DATE DUE

NOV 1 8 1993	
Dec 07 1993	
UPI SPO-125	PRINTED IN U.S.A.

THE TECHNOLOGY EXPLOSION IN MEDICAL SCIENCE:
Implications for the Health Care Industry and the Public (1981-2001)

Monographs in Health Care Administration
Series Editor, Samuel Levey, Ph.D., University of Iowa

Volume 1:

Competition in the Marketplace: Health Care in the 1980's
Edited by James R. Gay and Barbara J. Sax Jacobs

Volume 2:

The Technology Explosion in Medical Science: Implications
for the Health Care Industry and the Public (1981-2001)
Edited by James R. Gay and Barbara J. Sax Jacobs

The Technology Explosion in Medical Science: Implications for the Health Care Industry and the Public (1981-2001)

Edited by

James R. Gay, M.D.
Barbara J. Sax Jacobs, J.D.

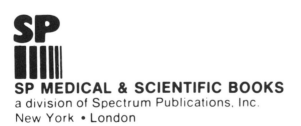

SP MEDICAL & SCIENTIFIC BOOKS
a division of Spectrum Publications, Inc.
New York • London

SPECTRUM PUBLICATIONS, INC.
175-20 Wexford Terrace, Jamacia, N.Y. 11432

Library of Congress Cataloging in Publication Data

Frank M. Norfleet Forum (2nd: 1981: University of
    Tennessee Center for the Health Sciences)
    The technology explosion in medical science.

    (Monographs in health care administration; v. 2)
    Bibliography: p.
    1. Medical innovations--Congresses. 2. Medical
innovations--Economic aspects--Congresses. I. Gay,
James R.   II. Jacobs, Barbara J. Sax. III. Title.
IV. Series. [DNLM: 1. Technology assessment, Biomedical
--Congresses. 2. Technology--Trends--Congresses.
3. Delivery of health care--Trends--Congresses.
4. Medicine--Trends--Congresses. W1 MO567N v. 2/W 84.1
T255 1981]
R856.A2F7 1981   338.4'5613621'0973   82-16763
ISBN 0-89335-181-4

The Frank Norfleet Forum
for the Advancement of Health

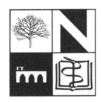

THE UNIVERSITY OF TENNESSEE
CENTER FOR THE HEALTH SCIENCES

EDITORIAL STAFF

James R. Gay, M.D., Editor
Director of Special Programs
The University of Tennessee
Center for the Health Sciences

Barbara J. Sax Jacobs, J.D., Editor
Research Associate (Administrative)
Office of the Vice Chancellor for
Academic Affairs
The University of Tennessee
Center for the Health Sciences

Cynthia B. Kent, Administrative Secretary
Office of Special Programs
The University of Tennessee
Center for the Health Sciences

ACKNOWLEDGMENT

The Office of the Norfleet Forum consists of the director and an administrative secretary who devote a substantial part of their time toward planning and coordinating this annual event. The efforts of a large number of volunteers who are university employees is necessary for successful production of the Norfleet Forum.

Chancellor James C. Hunt, M.D., the Trustees, and numerous individual faculty and staff members serving on small task forces assisted the director in designing the format, defining the content and selecting the participants. The Director is grateful for all persons who contributed ideas, time and effort to all aspects of the forum process.

Barbara Sax Jacobs and Cynthia Brock Kent assumed major responsibility for editing the proceedings and preparing the final manuscript. Their dedication to this important task was exceptional.

The contributors to this volume are representative of a small group of elite thinkers who provide an inexhaustable well of ideas needed for solving the most pressing of the socio-economic problems of the nation. The Director is grateful for their generosity in preparing the content of the Forum and assisting in the completion of the proceedings.

The Trustees thank Dunbar Abston, Sr., Frank and Jean Norfleet, Norfleet Turner, Sam H. Sanders, M.D., Sam Cooper, and Texas Gas Transmission for the contributions that support the Norfleet Forum. Mr. Maurice Ancharoff and the staff of Spectrum Publications, Incorporated are cited by the Editors for their exceptional interest and cooperation.

CONTRIBUTORS

H. David Banta, M.D., M.P.H.
Assistant Director
United States Congress
Office of Technology Assessment
Washington, D.C.

Theodore Cooper, M.D., Ph.D.
Executive Vice President
The Upjohn Company
Kalamazoo, Michigan

Ruth S. Hanft
Senior Research Associate
Association of Academic Health Centers
Washington, D.C.

Clark C. Havighurst, J.D.
Professor of Law
Duke University
Durham, North Carolina

Stephen C. Joseph, M.D., M.P.H.
Chief of Pediatrics, Locum Tenens
Grenfell Regional Health Services
St. Anthony, Newfoundland
Canada

J. Michael McGinnis, M.D., M.P.P.
Deputy Assistant Secretary for Health
and Assistant Surgeon General
Department of Health and Human Services
Washington, D.C.

Robert H. Moser, M.D., F.A.C.P.
Executive Vice President
American College of Physicians
Philadelphia, Pennsylvania

Arnold S. Relman, M.D.
Editor
New England Journal of Medicine
Boston, Massachusetts

Benson B. Roe, M.D.
Professor of Surgery
University of California
San Francisco, California

J. Michael Schiffer
Director of Group Insurance Government Relations
Connecticut General Life Insurance Company
Hartford, Connecticut

Milton C. Weinstein, Ph.D.
Professor of Policy and Decision Sciences
Harvard School of Public Health
Boston, Massachusetts

FOREWORD

The second annual Frank M. Norfleet Forum for the Advancement of Health was convened November 30, December 1 and 2, 1981 at The University of Tennessee Center for the Health Sciences, Memphis, Tennessee.

The Norfleet Forum is a continuing series of discussions on issues related to national health policy and organization of health care at all levels.

Application of the competitive model for containing costs and assuring high quality of medical care (1980 Forum) is jeopardized in part by rapid introduction of expensive medical technology.

Decision-makers in business and industry, government and health care provider groups recognize the benefits of high technology and are reluctant to impose controls that might reduce the effective level of scientific creativity.

And yet, some technologies are rushed into routine use before their efficacy and safety are assured, and without measuring the benefits to be achieved against the harsh reality of cost.

In this volume, 11 of the world's experts on technology issues summarize current ideas for understanding and coping with the technological imperative of the 1980s.

James R. Gay, M.D.
Director, The Norfleet Forum

TABLE OF CONTENTS

I.   The Status of Medical Care: 1
        Where We Are and Where We Are Going
        Theodore Cooper

II.   The Intellectual Imperative and   17
        The New Technology
        Robert H. Moser

III.   Iron Axe, Magic Lamp, or Trojan Horse: 33
        Issues in Cross-Cultural Transfer of
        Health Technology
        Stephen C. Joseph

IV.   Economic Impact and Cost-Effectiveness 47
        of Medical Technology
        Milton C. Weinstein

V.   Competition and Health Care Technology 71
        Can We Decentralize Decision Making?
        Clark C. Havighurst

VI.   Some Aphorisms Concerning Medical Technology 85
        Illustrated by Specific Case Examples
        H. David Banta

VII.   Technology Assessment By Physicians   101
        Arnold S. Relman

VIII.   Physician Remuneration: 111
        Boondoggle or Bust?
        Benson B. Roe

IX.   Monitoring Medical Technology: 121
        Shall Technology Be Regulated?
        How and By Whom?
        Ruth S. Hanft

X.   Reimbursement for Technology: 135
        The Insurer's Dilemma
        H. Michael Schiffer

XI.   Allocating Resources for Health   143
        J. Michael McGinnis

        Appendix A: Forum Trustees and   155
        University President

THE STATUS OF MEDICAL CARE: WHERE WE ARE AND WHERE WE ARE GOING
Theodore Cooper, M.D.

I begin with an assertion. Medical care in this country is good, very good, and it is going to get better because there is a dynamic system of research feeding into the system that which is necessary for improvement--knowledge and information.

Is medical care everything that everyone wants it to be? Surely the answer is no. Does that mean that medical care is poor? Not to my way of thinking. People usually want different things when they characterize the status of American medicine. Note that I said want, not need. "Wants" become "needs" with dazzling speed these days.

Some people want the system to go beyond its current technical capabilities. Some want a better quality of professionalism. Some want access, particularly to a higher standard of care. Some want greater amenities. Some want greater convenience. Some want more personalized attention. Some want more understanding of what is proposed to be done or what has been done. Others want guaranteed re-sults. But many want whatever it is they are getting for less cost. Most people believe that health care costs too much.

Basically, everyone wants vigor, vitality, immunity from the consequences of self-abuse, and longevity. Unfortu-nately, we have acquired the notion that these wants can be bought on demand from or through physicians or from some-one else in the system.

Is it any wonder, then, that discussions about health programs and policies often lapse into enumerations of shortcomings in the absence of any agreed-upon set of values? Deficiencies become problems; rhetoric focuses on the negative. The public is convinced that something is wrong, but they are not sure what it is. There is melancholia mixed with melodrama.

Have we temporarily lost our sanity? In health-related matters, it seems that we have. We are having trouble seeing a forest of constructive change and fantastic opportunity for the trees of rising costs and unwieldy programs. Being too absorbed in costs and cost savings can color one's perspective and can make it difficult to take an objective look at the system of medical care in this country and its future.

There is a frantic negativism running around loose in America. Americans are absorbed in the word "crisis." In the health care field, there is the Medicare crisis, the malpractice crisis, the hospital-cost crisis, the quality crisis, and the nursing crisis.

An instructive way to look at crisis might result from thinking about the Chinese word for crisis. Their word comprises two symbols: "danger" on the top, and "opportunity" on the bottom. This view of the word holds that there is an element of danger in crisis, and there are undoubtedly dangers facing medical care in this country. But it also holds that danger says that something is being done wrong. Therefore, crisis gives someone the opportunity to step back and look at himself, to redirect his thinking, and to take advantage of a changing world.

It is the opportunities, then, that I find so intriguing as I look at the status of medicine in the United States. My strongest sense about the future is that we will be carried there by winds of change. These winds blow from the direction of economics, quality, technology, and attitudes. Economists prowl the inner circles of public policymaking these days, and that is probably why so much attention is paid to the volume of dollars spent on health in this country. There is no doubt that the rate of increase in these costs, more than 15 percent last year, must be checked. Still, when you consider the billions of dollars spent on health, you should recognize that there are great opportunities to accomplish things, not only that a lot of money is being spent.

There is also a great deal of concern about the quality

of medical care in this country.   Some say it is too high, given third-party reimbursement.   Others say it is too low, given the fact that between 22 million and 25 million Americans have no health insurance.   Mind you, I said health insurance not health care.   These questions about quality are important, and they give us a chance to realize that too often we have looked at the statistics of programs rather than at the performance of the delivery system itself.   I think we have the opportunity to change the system of delivering medical care to the point where every citizen can receive medical care of adequate quality with reasonable accessibility. Mind you, I did not say that everyone should get or could get the same care or equal care.

For me, technology is a great spring of optimism.   The work being done now in laboratories around the world in areas such as surface chemistry, immunology, genetics, neurosciences, behavioral sciences, receptor theory, and biology--just to mention a few--will soon broaden the scope of medicine far beyond what was imagined possible only a few years ago.

We must be careful, however, to avoid being swept away by this tide of technological innovation, and must realize that technology carries with it important questions. How and where will new technology be applied? Who will apply it? Who will pay for it?   Should all the latest technology filter down to every community hospital, or should it be contained in regional centers? If these questions are answered intelligently, public policy and medical innovation should be able to work together for a change.

Figure 1 indicates how health care expenditure money is spent.   Note that hospitals and nursing homes account for nearly 50 percent of the total bill.   Other costs, such as physicians, drugs, and dentists are also clearly delineated, but the "other" category, which accounts for a relatively large amount of money, is less specific.   These monies are not directly associated with patient care and therefore are available for application to medical-social problems and to problem solving.

The increases in health care expenditures during this past year derive from more than just price inflation, although that accounts for 60 percent of the increase.   There is some expansion due to greater intensity of care, which flows usually from technology or from the perceived reasons to use it, and also from expanding the base of the population that will be served. I am not sure that we should be surprised that the rate of expansion of expenditures in the health care sector, therefore, exceeds the consumer price index. (Figure 2). It is more than just price inflation, labor costs, supplies costs.

Direct individual payments are becoming a lesser percentage of payments in the system, while government payments are rising. Private health insurance, which is funded largely by employers, is still rising. (Figure 3). And it is important to note that these employers are becoming concerned. They are demanding better data from insurance carriers. They are analyzing hospital data more critically to see where the money is being spent. They are trying to determine whether their health insurance monies are being effectively and efficiently used. And, many employers and carriers now subscribe to experiments in cost reduction or cost containment in programs such as mandatory or voluntary second opinions.

Forty-two percent of the health bill is paid by the public purse--the federal, state, and local governments. (Figure 4). Is it any wonder that the leverage of public sources is increasing to where they follow the golden rule, that he who has the gold makes the rules? We as a nation now spend more than $1,000 per capita for our health care. (Figure 5).

It is against this background that Americans hear they may be asking for too much from the health care system, particularly too much from the public purse. The current administration feels this increasing reliance on the federal portion of the public expenditures is wrong. An administration spokesman said not too long ago that Americans cannot afford to fund the Great Society any longer; the great expansion in health care costs was part of the original Great Society thrust.

The early changes in federal health policy are supposed to allow more local definition of health care needs and of the methods employed to meet those needs. Research incentives are contained in the new tax bill. More preventive medicine programs are being encouraged through local employers and local agencies, including state and county health departments. They are being encouraged, though not necessarily funded, with new federal dollars. That is not to say that there are no strong moves at the federal level to change the methods of overall financing of health care or for the es-

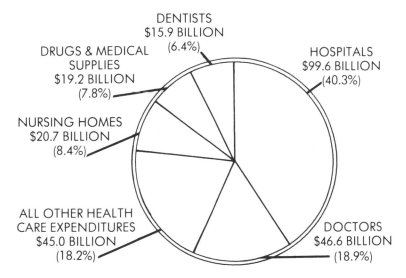

NOTE: 36% of all hospital expenditures were attributable to Medicare/Medicaid

Figure 1. How the U.S. spent $247 billion on health care in 1980

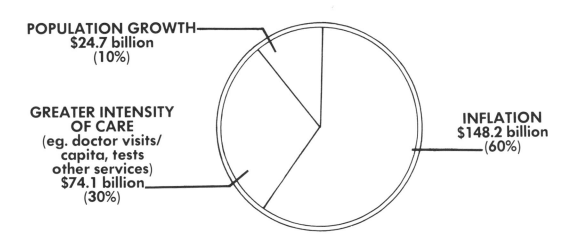

Figure 2. 1980 U.S. health care costs increased 15.2% over 1979 to $247 billion

Percent of all health care expenditures

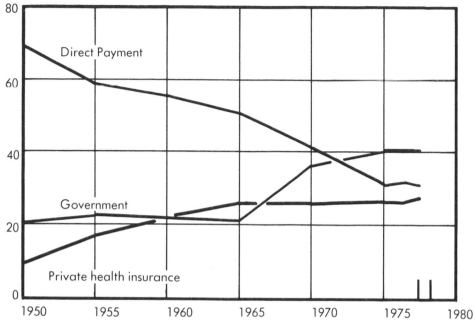

Figure 3. National and personal expenditures for health care, by source of payment, selected years - 1950 - 1977.

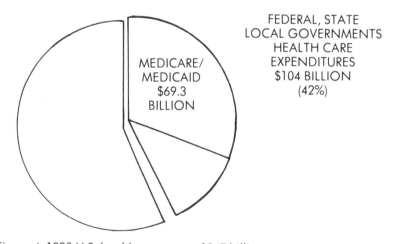

Figure 4. 1980 U.S. health care costs $247 billion

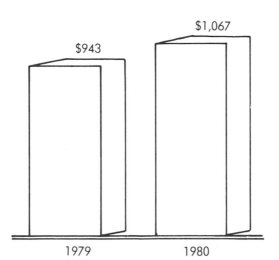

Figure 5. U.S. per capita health care costs

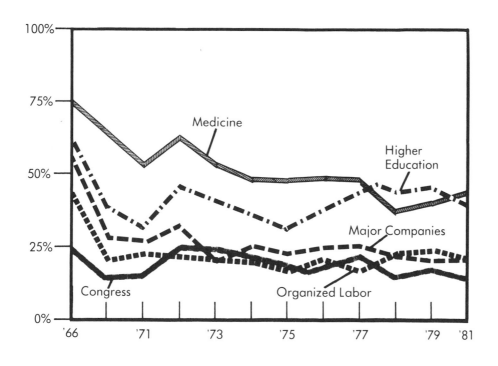

Figure 6. Confidence in the leaders of institutions. The Harris Survey

tablishment of accountability standards. The usual array of task forces are at work in Washington. They are focusing on what is known as competition, as was discussed at the Norfleet Forum last year. Their use of competition, in my view, will not succeed, because it ignores the traditional American value placed on health. It asks the wrong people to make important choices, and therefore it is unlikely to be endorsed by any constituency large enough to ensure passage.

Not only Medicaid caps, but Medicare caps also, are likely in the future. These caps will be fought vigorously because such caps take into consideration only the amount of money that is pumped into the system, and not how the system actually makes use of that money.

The effects of the changes in federal health policy are as follows:

1. More local initiative and emphasis.

2. Employers initiating preventive programs.

3. Research incentives through taxes and regulatory shifts.

4. Federal establishment and local implementation of large-scale public health programs.

Comprehensive national insurance remains of interest, but the monies that would be needed to establish such a program are so politically impossible at this time that serious discussion of such a program is not feasible.

There are changing perceptions about health concerns. One of the most important changes is what the public thinks is important. The following data come from a recent Yankelovich poll:

"How Much Concern Do Americans Show About Their Health As Compared to Several Years Ago?"

MORE CONCERN	70% Agree
LESS CONCERN	12% Agree
ABOUT THE SAME	18% Agree

Obviously, more Americans care more about their health as compared to several years ago. Because of attitudes such as this, any decisions made on controls, limitations, and cutbacks in service must take into account the high value placed on health by the American citizen. And this is one big reason why it will be so difficult for the public policy change based on notions of cutback in health care to succeed. The American public has virtually accepted the idea, philosophically, that--for their health care--more is better.

Americans, therefore, might accept one of the following propositions, or they might accede to what is already in law in Public Law 93-641, the Health Planning Act, that every citizen should have access to quality care at reasonable cost. But health care is seen by many people in this country as a right. In my view, the goal should be quality care that is reasonably accessible, not a single class of care because if we try to establish a single class of care and standardize quality in that way, such standardization usually occurs at the bottom. It is a minimum standard. The first level of challenge, therefore, is to provide a core of professional services that are not standardized at the bottom of the quality scale and priced at the top of the cost scale.

There is another kind of change that is occurring in our system, and that concerns the confidence that our citizens have in our various institutions in society. Although medicine has enjoyed a substantial decline, the public still expects a great deal from the profession, more than from any other institution. And physicians are as respected as leaders of any other institution, or more so. It is interesting to note there is a distinct air of pessimism that can be traced back 10 or 15 years. Thus, expectations and trust do not necessarily go hand in hand. (Figure 6).

Relaxation of regulations is currently another theme of change; however, in the health field the specifics remain to be defined. But if regulation really declines in the health care field, and I am not at all sure that it will, public scrutiny will increase.

Quality becomes a self-preservation issue under these kinds of evaluation systems. Many questions will have to be dealt with, including such things as the mandated use of allied health professionals, and changes in licensure laws and record keeping. Regulation by way of media exposure will occur and will be uncomfortable for most.

We often discuss the need for change as if no change in the structure of the system itself were occurring. But indeed there are many significant modifications going on rapidly right now in the system. One new trend in health care and health care financing as indicated in Figure 7 has been the increase in the number of for-profit hospitals. These privately owned hospitals show that some people are rethinking ways to finance health care. If privately owned hospitals are to be more than acute care centers for the wealthy or easy treatment centers, more thought needs to be directed toward how hospital resources are used. There is no doubt that the character of all these resources will be changing rapidly. Same-day care in hospitals, ambulatory centers, educational centers, and rehabilitation centers will become more and more a part of our hospitals. The in-patient preoccupation of the last 15 years will change, provided we have enough foresight, insight and courage to properly change the incentive system.

The public is also driving at other changes. Attached to all the debate about changes in the quality and the status of the system is the problem of litigation. To me it seems that litigation has put too much rigidity in the system. Perhaps discussions with the legal profession about fault and outcomes of care need to be intensified to make attorneys more realistic about what is possible and honest and fair.

There are other kinds of forces driving the core of our activities. Just as the public's estimation of the physician has decreased, so, too, has the credibility of scientists decreased. (Figure 8).

Regarding change, Figure 9 illustrates some interesting health statistics and points out where attention needs to be directed in the future. One should not conclude that the changes illustrated are all the result of the performance of the medical system as improvement in the standard of living has probably made a greater contribution to these changes.

One can get a good idea of the magnitude of the change that has taken place by comparing the causes of death in 1978 against those in 1900. Important public health problems, such as arthritis and other debilitating diseases often associated with a longer-lived population, need to be addressed. We must learn to deal with an aging population because it will be another opportunity to do more things better for more people. We now have the chance to take geriatric medicine beyond treating symptoms of chronic dis-

Total Number: 6,000

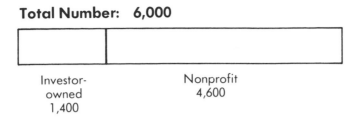

Investor-
owned
1,400

Nonprofit
4,600

Number of Beds: 1,000,000

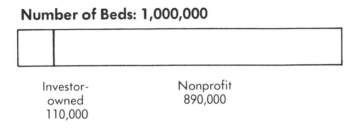

Investor-
owned
110,000

Nonprofit
890,000

Figure 7. Community hospitals - 1981

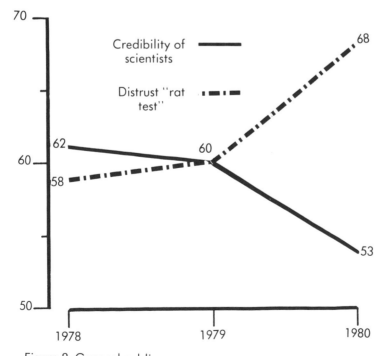

Figure 8. General public

1900 (Total: 1779/100,000)

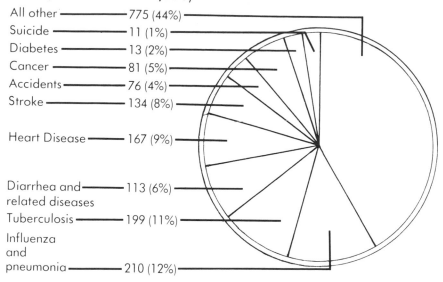

All other ——————775 (44%)——————
Suicide ——————11 (1%)——————
Diabetes ——————13 (2%)——————
Cancer ——————81 (5%)——————
Accidents——————76 (4%)——————
Stroke——————134 (8%)——————

Heart Disease——————167 (9%)——————

Diarrhea and——————113 (6%)——————
related diseases
Tuberculosis——————199 (11%)——————
Influenza
and
pneumonia——————210 (12%)——————

1978 (Total: 606/100,000)

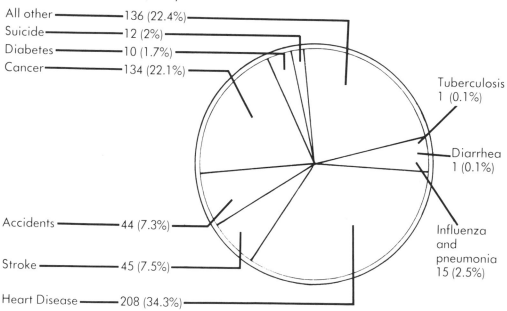

All other ——————136 (22.4%)——————
Suicide——————12 (2%)——————
Diabetes——————10 (1.7%)——————
Cancer——————134 (22.1%)——————

Tuberculosis
1 (0.1%)

Diarrhea
1 (0.1%)

Accidents ——————44 (7.3%)——————

Influenza
and
pneumonia
15 (2.5%)

Stroke ——————45 (7.5%)——————

Heart Disease ——————208 (34.3%)——————

Figure 9. Leading causes of death in 1900 and 1978.

Overall age adjusted death rate per 100,000 for the leading causes of death in 1900 compared with 1978.

Numbers in parentheses indicate percentages of total age adjusted death rate.

eases and maintaining life for just an extra few years.

The key to the success of the performance of the medical care or health care system, whatever it may have contributed to that excellent overall performance, has been research. Research is still the most cost-effective and precise way to improve the nation's health. We are ushering in a new era or a new plateau in what is known as biotechnology. We shall learn more about cause. And with techniques evolving from such developments we shall be able to do something else: we shall be able to detect individuals who are susceptible to disease. This ability to detect susceptibility will take large-scale statistics and extrapolation out of the attempt to enfold preventive medicine back into the physician's hands. The physician will not have to guess. On the basis of population studies, he will have a background against which to ply an individual's specific data to determine when to effect the earliest possible intervention in an individual susceptible to any number of disease processes. This will lead to the creation of more precise, specific pharmaceuticals. It will also lead to a much-reduced exposure of individuals to the necessary clinical trials and, indeed, will reduce the cost of research and the clinical trials themselves, a very important set of evolving developments.

There are yet other changes in what can be done. We often think that people pay insufficient attention to all of the admonitions about diet. But there are many changes in health practices occurring among the U.S. population. Americans are moving away from diets high in animal fats, and there are some who feel that this will reduce cardiovascular problems. There is a generally increasing acceptance of the need to reduce sedentary living, resulting in an increased interest in exercise programs. Trends such as these, and the reduction in smoking in most segments of the population, must be encouraged not only by public officials or educators but also by the entire medical community. Prevention has become more than a shibboleth; the approaches are gradually gaining credence with the professionals as well as with the populace.

The understanding of how to improve prevention, based on sound scientific information regarding cause and susceptibility, will make a big change in this spectrum of data. Up until the present, the medical system performance has only been able to contribute about 10 percent to the reduction in mortality pointed out previously. Now as our standard of living stabilizes, we can expect to increase our intervention and continue our progress. Through the medical and health care system we will be able to effect the four things that make up 90 percent of the factors involved in prevention: Life-style (48 percent); Hereditary (biological) Factors (26 percent); Environment (16 percent); Medical System (10 percent).

Medical education itself is a form of technology but it has not kept pace with the other parts of medical technology. Our culture changes, and our way of practice in medicine changes, and we have gone through more and more specialization. Our problem is not that we have gone to specialization, but that we have been a little too narrow-minded about what specialization can do. Specialization can improve prevention as well as acute care. We have the opportunity to move towards educating what used to be known as the complete physician.

It is asserted by many that 9.4 percent of the gross national product is too much to be spent on health care. It is expected that this percentage, in fact, will increase. There is fanciful thinking that elimination of fraud or peer review or planning systems will help. Or that consensus reviews or technology assessment will save enough money to allow the remainder of activities to proceed without modification. I do not believe that such measures will have enough impact soon enough.

The pressures to reduce cost without sacrificing quality will necessitate changes, rapid changes, of a more profound nature. One radical suggestion has been to reduce our research significantly so that technology will not force new expenditures. I hope that we will not fall prey to such Luddite views.

Another suggestion has been to federalize the entire system, including fees and licensure. I hope we shall not fall victim to such frustration and expect that the federal government will be able to solve all our difficult problems. Its track record is not that good.

It is not enough, however, to reject all suggestions just because we do not agree with a philosophy or because we perceive weaknesses in the argument. What is needed is courage. Courage to recognize that there are limits. Limits to what we can expect from even this magnificent technology. Limits to what we should ask others to do for us. Limits to what is available to spend and, therefore, limits even to what should be charged. We need the courage to realize that the freedom to choose poorly is neither dignity nor quality and that the freedom to serve selectively, without price restraint, is not the essence of a professional.

This country's greatest resource is the health of its people. Research and technology will assure continued opportunities to build that resource. The turbulent, tedious, chaotic mechanisms of democracy will sort out ways to get these fantastic new things and those reliable old things to all of the people. We must believe it. It is the first requirement of success.

THE INTELLECTUAL IMPERATIVE AND THE NEW TECHNOLOGY
Robert H. Moser, M.D.

Among the many features that set Homo sapiens apart from his hominid brethren, one emerges preeminent. I have chosen to call it, the "intellectual imperative." It is the unquenchable spirit and relentless desire to explore and expand knowledge to the ultimate, to invent the uninvented, to discover the undiscovered, to create the uncreated. And devil take the consequences.

No power on earth can stop the mind of man. In science and in art, the single-minded dedication to pursuit of truth most often casts aside or ignores all external considerations; we call it purity of purpose. It is a magnificently naive concept. Naivete becomes the hand-maiden of purity. They travel together. The cynic may say this is a contrived liaison, but the scientist hot on the trail of new knowledge, most frequently, is not inclined to reckon with the social or political or economic implications of his potential discovery. The scientist, imprisoned in the grasp of the intellectual imperative, wears blinders.

I know of no instance in which the progress of science has stopped because of political or social or economic pressures. Many times it has been slowed or diverted, but eventually the work goes on as inexorably as the tides.

Splitting the atom was the ultimate expression of the intellectual imperative. Admittedly, the Manhattan Project was accelerated by momentous historical events, but many scientists were fascinated by the chase, per se. For them the potential for a nuclear Armageddon was thrust aside as a momentary dark reflection. It was late in the course of events when the conscience-pressured scientists wrote to

17

President Roosevelt and expressed their grave concern. The creation of the world's most horrendous weapons system was the result of an exciting progression of events: a concordance of theoretical mathematics and physics culminating in an avalanche of knowledge which dominated all external considerations. Nuclear weaponry has resurfaced as a major moral and political conundrum in this comparatively more contemplative, yet still anxious, period of world history. But the Manhattan Project remains as the transcendant incident in physical science; in one step it freed us from the constraints of Newtonian thinking and delivered us unto the limitless era of Einstein and quantum mechanics. And it was done with few sidelong glances.

In a similar vein, a like phenomenon is occurring in genetic engineering. The scientists who entered the fearsome lists of hybrid creativity paused only momentarily to reflect on the social, moral, and political implications. Then they cast out the demons of Andromeda and plunged ahead in their relentless pursuit of new biologic forms.

Now the research is continuing with unprecedented rapidity. Efforts are abroad to sever all regulatory restraints. A few nervous religious ethicists continue to scratch their heads in concern, but their voices are distant and timorous. I suspect that even if those anxious individuals who band together to articulate social concerns and those others who shape our legislation had ever joined forces to create laws to inhibit genetic engineering, the intellectual imperative would have prevailed; the laws would have been circumvented or violated, and the research would have continued.

Are we far removed from the clandestine anatomists of the Middle Ages who snatched still-warm bodies from the fresh green turf to explore the miracle of human anatomy, despite personal jeopardy to eye, limb, and life? The technological revolution we are experiencing today is only the most recent manifestation of the intellectual imperative. Thus the new technology--child of the nuclear-electronic age--is here, because it is time.

We can tether the giant of technology, but we cannot stop his growth. We can create laws to limit the production of H-bombs, but we cannot inhibit the research that explores and refines the theoretical underpinnings.

We can create laws to restrict applied research and limit

the varieties of hybridomas we intend to create, but we cannot inhibit the progression and technical refinement of genetic manipulation.

We can slow new technology by applying economic and political sanctions, but we will never stop the inspired investigator bewitched by the intellectual imperative. He will defy politics and economics and threats of physical harm. He will work in basements and garrets. He will plead for or purloin equipment to pursue his star. Once enmeshed, he is never released during the interval of creative intellectual activity. He is Galileo; he is Da Vinci; she is Curie. And in their hearts and minds they sing of art and science, and to others they whisper: "We give you this marvelous new thing; it is for you to control and exploit. We have no time for your puny politics or social concerns or economic gynmastics; it is for you to transmute this gold of knowledge into your baser metals of utility."

And I say it is good that we have today's wondrous tools in medicine. Our craft was never easier for practitioners or more effective for patients. In the not too distant past, making the diagnosis too often benefitted only the physicians intellectual ego; it mattered little to the patient. Even if the deductive exercise of diagnosis were successful, there was little physicians could offer. This is no longer the case. We understand the pathophysiology and mechanisms of disease as never before. We have diagnostic tools and therapeutic devices that are specific and effective.

Consequently, practitioners of medicine have never been more laden with responsibility. We have enormous unprecedented capability to help people, and we must become absolute masters of these tools. To do less is to break faith with our patients, to possibly deny them relief and cure.

The products of the medical intellectual imperative, both ideal and concrete, will continue to cascade from the ever-widening mouth of the cornucopia, and almost every one will be used ultimately, in some constructive and/or destructive philosophy or device.

But, as regards medical technology and pharmacology, we physicians are the "emptors" who must cry "caveat." We cannot afford, like Edmond Hillary, to scale the Everest of technology just "because it is there." And so we have a problem.

A host of crucial questions posed by the technology boom now face the profession. They can all be boiled down to several key issues. (1) How do you tether this magnificent giant? (2) Who shall control this vast new universe of biomedical technology? (3) And how big a problem is it really?

Between 1969 and 1978 expenditures for personal health care in the United States rose by $110 billion, with about 30 percent of this increase attributed to the greater use of what has been loosely called "technology." Writing in The New England Journal of Medicine in 1979, Dr. Relman cited the now-famous 1978 statistics: between $12-14 billion was spent on laboratory tests in that year. These expenditures have been increasing at about 15 percent per year. For example, in 1978, $8 billion was spent on radiographic diagnostic procedures, $600 million on CT scanning alone; an additional $1 billion on coronary arteriography and coronary bypass procedures, and another $1 billion on hemodialysis. Remember that was 1978.

David Banta has written "Other industrialized countries have experienced rises as rapid or even more rapid," and cites confirming statistics.

The clinical deployment use of new diagnostic procedures has a doubling-time reminiscent of leukemia cells.

Many of us have expressed concern about the inclination of many of those pundits who lament the fiscal problems which attend new technology, to focus on the glamorous high price/per unit items, such as CT scans and hemodialysis, because many of us feel there should be equal interest in the "small-ticket," widely-used procedures. We have the suspicion that it is the less-than judicious, widespread use of these small-ticket technologies that has contributed, in a major, if insidious manner, to the skyrocketing price of diagnostic and therapeutic procedures.

Moloney and Rogers estimated that in 1973 the bill for one class of these small-ticket technologies, that is routine clinical laboratory tests, exceeded the sum of capital equipment purchases by all U.S. hospitals by some $400 million. The actual numbers were: $600 million spent on hospital capital equipment purchases, while $1 billion was spent on clinical laboratory tests.

As a corollary theme, there has been a major concern among some educators in medicine that young people are making career decisions on the basis of the economic yield that attends certain high technology specialties. My own experience indicates that this is not the case at present. There have always been some students who opted for the lucrative specialties, for the specific purpose of making money. Yet, I believe that most students of medicine select careers on the basis of intellectual challenge and the "fit" of the specialty with their own professional talent and aspirations. However, it is a sad commentary that all this may change as the level of the student's indebtedness becomes more burdensome, and may tip the balance as young clinician-investigators contemplate an increasingly uncertain career in research and teaching versus clinical practice.

There is no question concerning the reality of being able to increase income by adding procedures to one's repertoire. Moloney and Rogers quote a study that indicated how physicians can increase annual net income from $31,000 to $90,000 simply by adding a number of so called "readily defensible" procedures to their standard workup. We all know of instances where a colleague, who has taken a quickie course in flexible endoscopy or broncoscopy or treadmill stress testing has been able to augment income by providing this new service. The hazard of this seduction is obvious. How do we balance the actual need for such services against the temptation to increase income?

Well, there has been much discussion about "inequitable reimbursement" for cognitive services versus procedural services. It has become a truism in such discussions to cite the general internist who spends 45 minutes with a new patient, eliciting historical information, performing a physical examination and then discussing the problem with the patient and the family. He carefully targets his diagnostic laboratory procedures. In most places this will earn him $50 to $100. If the same physician sees the patient swiftly, takes a cursory history, does a brief physical examination and then schedules and performs a treadmill stress test or a colonoscopy, he may earn four to ten times the income for the comparable time. How do we compensate for intellectual activity? How much is it worth to pay for the decision not to do the treadmill stress test; not to do the colonoscopy? And how can we devise such a system--perhaps a medical version of the farm subsidy--a system of financial incentives not to plant cotton, or not to increase the herd.

In all candor, when one considers the average income of physicians, and I speak as one who has toiled in the vineyard of private practice, I would find it difficult to justify a position that contends we are under-reimbursed for intellectual activity, while remaining silent on the point of possible overcompensation for procedural activities. Reimbursement is a two-way street, and the traffic must flow in both directions. Compensation for medical services is a sticky wicket, but it is an area we must study, and I suspect, rather soon.

Dr. Al Roberts, writing in the American College of Physicians Observer cites still another aspect of the technology conundrum. He said:

"Excessive reliance on and overpayment for tests and procedures erode the quality of medical practice. Physicians, hospitals and laboratories are all rewarded for testing. Physicians, and especially House Officers, may order a test 'to learn from it'--that is to say, to acquire experience in evaluating procedures in real life clinical settings. Whether this is, in fact, beneficial is questionable. Some harm is obvious: the loss or atrophy of the powers of parsimonious reasoning from critical observation; an unwillingness or inability to discriminate between what is central and what is ancillary in an illness; the decline of the arts of history taking and physical diagnosis; and the loss of the concept of testing as a scientific enterprise wherein the problem is first sharply defined as an hypothesis; to be tested by specific tests and orderly procedures, with a range of possible outcomes having been prospectively weighed in relation to treatment and prognosis. This is clinical reasoning at its best, the very heart and soul of internal medicine and a fundamental tradition of the American College of Physicians. It is time to reassert the central role of clinical reasoning."

Then there is another dimension to the technology conundrum.

There is no question that a great portion of the criticism that has been leveled at medicine is that clinicians have become mere extensions, willing slaves, if you will, to the glistening hardware that inhabits the clinical laboratory.

All of us old clinicians decry the fast shuffle that students and House Officers give to the soft, unquantifiable data of the subjective history, and the cumbersome, time consuming process of careful laying on of the hands--physical examination--in an effort to move quickly onto the terra firma of objectivity: the neatly typed numbers on clean white laboratory slips. We are all aware of the expanding universe of diagnostic capability that has come to our fingertips with the maturation of the clinical laboratory. But I share the fear that, at times, we have been overly charmed, in fact, hypnotized by the glistening creatures of the clinical laboratory, with the attendant erosion of bedside skills and clinical reasoning. Add to this the economic disincentives built into the system which reward procedural effort and you begin to perceive the magnitude and subtlety of the problem.

But we have drifted. What can we do to bring the proper use of these marvelous new tests and procedures into appropriate context? How can we be sure that they will be deployed with care and parsimony in keeping with our tradition of practicing lean, scientific medicine?

The problem has been addressed by many agencies including the National Center for Health Care Technology, the Office of Technology Assessment, the National Center for Health Services Research, the Food and Drug Administration, the National Institutes of Health, and the Health Care Financing Administration. In addition, the American College of Physicians (ACP) has several programs, one which is very exciting: the Clinical Efficacy Assessment Project (CEAP).

A major thrust of the College's effort is to help curb the cost of medical care in the United States without compromising quality. Realistically, the segments of the cost of medical care that are controlled directly by physicians are three: ordering patients into the hospitals; writing prescriptions; and ordering tests and procedures. Physicians have little or no direct control over cost of beds per day, cost of services, capital equipment purchases and of course inflation.

But we do believe that physicians must be more cost conscious. Experience with health maintenance organizations has indicated that hospital utilization rates decline when there are appropriate financial incentives. I do not think this is related to purposeful under-utilization--but rather to prudent use of hospital facilities. Careful, even parsimonious selection of diagnostic tests and judicious choice of therapeutic interventions is, indeed, in the finest tradition of clinical medicine, and fortunately, this thoughtful process is also cost effective.

It is almost a truism that many tests and procedures that served as tools in the past, when knowledge was more limited and technology more primitive, came into widespread clinical use with little scientific evidence of their worth. Some have proved to be ineffective and were abandoned. Still others have been superceded by newer, more reliable or more specific techniques that have evolved through advancement in our knowledge of chemistry, pathophysiology of disease and increased sophistication of laboratory tools. This progress caused most older procedures to fall by the wayside. But some tests and procedures persisted and became almost traditions, with little thought given to their shaky scientific origins or dubious clinical merit. We found that many such anachronistic tests and procedures were still being ordered. They contributed little or nothing to quality of care, but added considerably to the cost of care.

For these reasons, the American College of Physicians agreed, in 1976, to participate in the Medical Necessity Project, a conjoint effort with Blue Cross/Blue Shield. Later, the Health Insurance Association of America, the National Center for Health Care Technology, working on behalf of the Medicare branch of the Health Care Financing Administration, and a number of other organizations, joined in the effort to evaluate specific diagnostic and treatment modalities according to their scientific merit and, especially, their clinical utility. This joint endeavor was designed to review procedures in current clinical use, on the basis of the reasons I presented earlier.

For five years, this effort was accomplished successfully by reviewing relatively simple tests and procedures that were generally conceded to be worthless or obsolete. But no one had taken the trouble to say so--formally. The American College of Physicians' recommendations about the clinical effectiveness of specific tests were predicated on review of available literature, plus the sound clinical judgment of acknowledged experts (clinical pathologists, subspecialists, and working clinicians), since, quite often very little supporting literature could be found to substantiate the effectiveness of a test or procedure that had been used in clinical medicine for many years. At times, the absence of supporting data turned out to be a most revealing and distressing experience.

Thus far, with few exceptions, College recommendations have received widespread endorsement by the medical community. Coincidentally, a decline in ordering these tests and procedures by physicians has resulted in significant savings. For example, in 1976, the ACP recommended that phonocardiograms should not be reimbursed routinely except upon the presentation of scientifically valid, written justification. An evaluation of the Federal Employee Program claims data by Blue Cross/Blue Shield showed that phonocardiograms decreased by 42.3 percent from 1975 to 1978. There were 1,324 claims in 1975 and 759 claims in 1978. Extrapolation of these data to the entire U.S. population represented a savings of approximately $860,000, for just this one procedure. This was not aimed at proper deployment of phonocardiograms which, in many instances, is a most valuable asset in the diagnosis of specific cardiac diseases, but rather the indiscriminate use of the procedure, all too often incorporated as part of a routine examination.

However, the complexity and controversial nature of many recent tests and procedures being forwarded to the College for such review have increased. Extensive reliance on the judgment of experts was no longer acceptable as a sufficient mechanism to justify our recommendations. For the medical community, third-party payers, and the federal government to accept ACP assessment of scientific validity and clinical usefulness of tests and procedures, it was recognized that a more sophisticated method of investigation was required. For this reason, the College expanded into the Clinical Efficacy Assessment Project (CEAP).

In order to do it properly, the College went to the Hartford Foundation and requested a three-year grant to expand staff and capability. Hartford saw the advantage of having a major private sector organization participate in the process, and the grant was forthcoming.

The College is in the process of establishing a Physicians' Network that will bracket the country, utilizing some 3,000 to 5,000 College members who will function as clinical investigators in the field, providing an essential dimension of practical input into the evaluation process.

The CEAP is being geared up to undertake evaluation of new and emerging tests and procedures--once the current backlog is caught up. We are looking to the future when, perhaps, the CEAP Physician Network will represent an ongoing clinical research effort to do post marketing surveillance of drugs and devices. But we are far away from that at present.

The other major endeavor of the College in the effort to help tether the technology giant was to teach physicians a logical decision making technique in the selection and interpretation of diagnostic tests and procedures. This effort culminated in the production of a Supplement to the Annals of Internal Medicine, which was written by Dr. Paul Griner and his associates. In the preamble to the Supplement, Dr. Griner wrote:

"The process of diagnosis requires two essential steps. The first is the establishment of diagnostic hypotheses followed by attempts to reduce their number by progressively ruling out specific diseases. This process requires very sensitive tests. Such tests, when normal, permit the physician to confidently exclude the disease. The next step is the pursuit of a strong clinical suspicion. This process requires a very specific test. Such a test, when abnormal, should essentially confirm the presence of the disease.

"The intelligent selection of a laboratory test, thus depends upon a choice that is appropriate for the purpose intended.

"The other requirement is that the purpose accurately reflect the physician's estimate of the likelihood of disease based on his/her assessment of the available clinical information. The use of tests to exclude or to confirm a diagnosis should indeed indicate that the physician's best estimate, after a careful evaluation of the patient's problem, is that the diagnosis in question is either unlikely or probable respectively.

"When these principles are followed, the conclusions reached from laboratory test results are likely to be correct and lead to appropriate diagnostic or therapeutic decisions."

Thus, the Supplement is an educational handbook instructing the physician in the area of decision making with a carefully delineated algorithmic technique, emphasizing the use of concepts of disease probability, sensitivity, and specificity.   Over 120,000 copies of the Supplement have been distributed.   The College is now in the process of designing a protocol that will test the impact on physician behavior of different levels of exposure to the information contained in the Supplement.

Thus, in two major areas the College is intimately involved in bringing the new technologies to heel, and utilize them appropriately in the practice of clinical medicine.

Another critical aspect of the technology conundrum is the expression of concern relating to the obligation of physicians to retain control.   To quote Dr. Al Roberts, "Imagine a scenario radically different from the familiar one.   What would happen if the rules of medical practice were relaxed to enlarge the domain of nurse practitioners, psychologists, physicians' assistants, social workers, chiropractors, podiatrists, nutritionists, and others to include access to hospitals, laboratories, and procedures? What if we had prescribing pharmacists as well?   The consequences would be hard to assess; they go to the heart of the meaning and purposes of a learned profession."

Roberts' concern is related to clinical judgment--that elusive aspect of medicine that is often lost in the swirling considerations of competition, practice patterns and patient expectations.   He focuses on use of the clinical laboratory.   It takes many years of study and experience to develop clinical judgment.   Those who lack this essential talent, are apt to be insecure and lack discrimination in their earnest zeal not to miss important medical problems. "I submit," he writes, "that the consequences would be mischief and confusion.   More testing, more errors in interpretation, and vastly increased expense.   This would be quite opposite what the FTC says it intended when it refers to the 'free marketplace.'   The only restraining mechanism apart from ultimate sheer weight of expense, is the well trained physician--who exercises clinical judgment."

Thus, I would defend medicine's continued control over biomedical technology.

Indeed, as we grapple with ways to contain and utilize the new technologies, I am reminded of a bit of wisdom mixed with whimsy that was written by Lewis Thomas in his Lives of a Cell that helps keep things in perspective. He wrote about the problem of new and emerging technologies.

"My suggestion for a new way to develop answers is to examine, in detail, the ways in which the various parts of todays medical care technology are used, from one day to the next, by the most sophisticated, knowledgable, and presumably satisfied consumers who now have full access to the system--namely, the well-trained, experienced, middle-aged, married-with-family internists.

"I could design the questionnaire, I think. How many times in the past five years have the members, including yourself, had any kind of laboratory tests? How many complete physical examinations? X-rays? Electrocardiograms? How often, in a years turning, have you prescribed antibiotics of any kind for yourself or your family? How many hospitalizations? How much surgery? How many consultations with a psychiatrist? How many formal visits to a doctor, including yourself? I will bet..." Thomas continues, "that if you got this kind of information, and added everything up, you will find a quite different set of figures from the ones now being projected in official circles for the population at large. I have tried it already, in an unscientific way, by asking around among my friends. My data, still soft but fairly consistent, reveals that none of my internist friends have had a routine physical examination since military service; very few have been x-rayed except by dentists; almost all have resisted surgery; laboratory tests for anyone in the family are extremely rare. They use a lot of aspirin, but they seem to write very few prescriptions and almost never treat family fever with antibiotics. This is not to say that they do not become ill; these families have the same incidence of chiefly respiratory and gastrointestinal illnesses as everyone else, and the same number of anxieties and bizarre notions, and the same number--on balance--a small number--of frightening or devastating diseases...

"The great secret known to internists and learned early in marriage by internists' wives, but still hidden from the general public, is that

most things get better by themselves.   Most
things, in fact, are better by morning."

And we know this is true.   Internists who we consider
to be among the more sophisticated of medical practitioners,
are extraordinarily parsimonious with the use of diagnostic
tests, procedures and drugs when it comes to themselves and
members of their own family, and yet they have the easiest
access to such things of any comparable group.

There is a major lesson to be learned here, and it is
related to sophistication, to appreciating the very real
limitations of medicine, of knowing of the natural history
of symptoms and signs--detecting those herald diseases that
are self-limited--and those that presage more ominous illness.   It also includes a profound appreciation of the
potential adverse effects of diagnostic tests and procedures
and drugs.

So, to summarize.   How can this great, new, pervasive
capability that has come about through the explosion in
technology be controlled?

First, through physician education.   One hears a lot
about so-called "pressure" to perform tests--evolved through
fear of litigation, and "pressure" to remain current because
of the increasing sophistication of patients who read popular magazines.   And this is laden on to the natural insecur-
ity of the conscientious clinician--who does not want to err
in diagnosis or treatment.

Physicians must resist these external pressures.   This
reinforcement can be facilitated through Professional Standards Review Organizations or a similar peer review mechanism in which national standards are published, which protect the physician who selects his tests and procedures and
drugs with care and circumspection.   The ACP will help
through careful evaluation of clinical effectiveness of
tests and procedures; indicating those that are worthless
or outdated.   Physicians must be reinforced in the simple
syllogism that clear indications, based on firm data, serve
as an invaluable foundation for the use of new tests, procedures and drugs.   Thus armed they should feel secure from
threat of litigation or fear of public pressure, and confident in their ability to make clinical decisions.

Second, there must be public education.   The people
must be instructed about the limitations, as well as the ca-

pabilities, of medicine. They must learn that each week does not produce wonder tests, wonder drugs, wonder diets, wonder results. This could be facilitated by an enlightened medical press that would seek to educate the public about individual and collective self-help to prevent disease. They should exert peer pressure on colleagues who seek the sensational story that tends to raise false expectations through descriptions of breakthrough discoveries and magic cures. Some basic understanding of the way medicine works--explanation of scientific method versus anecdote, and always--the mission of medicine--primium non vocere. This would go a long way to facilitate a better utilization of medical technology.

Third, there must be a revision of our program of financial incentives and disincentives. We must decide once and for all, whether we are clever enough to devise a system that will reward for intellectual effort. In some way can the decision not to use the new technology, not to do the colonoscopy, not to do the treadmill stress test be rewarded? Are intellectual efforts being appropriately rewarded?

And, on the other hand, it is time for a hard-nosed study of reward for procedures; are some over-reimbursed?

In other words, there must be some balance in reimbursement; some reward system that will make it economically worthwhile to deploy tests, procedures and drugs in a rational, properly indicated fashion.

And, finally, we must rid ourselves--expunge--from our thinking the magic allure of the "Gadget Syndrome." I will never understand why so many physicians feel impelled to be trendy, to use the new test, procedure, or drug because it is au courant, because it is widely-publicized in advertisements, by patients and in the press--before it has passed the rigorous hurdles of scientific testing.

Each of these four items represents an essential integer in bringing America's marvelous, new technological advances into rational context.

I return to my previous thesis that we should not fear these new devices; we should respect them for the wonderful things they are, and rejoice for the remarkable benefits they can bring to the ill. And we must apply common sense and learn their strengths and weaknesses.

We must take them gently from the wizards who created them, and we must employ them with wisdom and sensitivity. Never in the past have we been able to do so much for so many.   And never has the responsibility been so great.

IRON AXE, MAGIC LAMP, OR TROJAN HORSE: ISSUES IN CROSS-CULTURAL TRANSFER OF HEALTH TECHNOLOGY

Stephen C. Joseph, M.D., M.P.H.

There is a traditional story among anthropologists that concerns an aboriginal tribe in Australia visited by Europeans for the first time. Upon their departure, the scientists left behind, as a gift, an iron axe. This was done with the best of motives, for clearly the product of modern technology was far superior to the less effective, less durable, and laboriously hand-crafted stone age implements made by the tribe. Unfortunately, the scientists had not taken into account the important social, political, and economic roles that the getting, making, trading, and using of stone axes played in that culture. The stone axe had important implications for rites of passage, for balance of economic power, for social status, and for tradition and ritual. The story goes on to detail the unraveling of a culture, in large part because of the "technologic transfer" of an iron axe.

The "iron axe" perspective is one that is often applied to the transfer of technology across cultural frontiers in our own time, especially with regard to the transfers between affluent and developing countries, between "modern" (post-industrial) and "traditional" (usually subsistence agricultural) communities, between what has come to be called "North" and "South."

Two other perspectives on this issue of technology transfer are commonly encountered; I choose to call them the "magic lamp" and the "Trojan horse." The original magic lamp was, of course, that marvel of technology acquired by Alladin, who had only (once he learned how to program it) to rub its sides, wait for the genie to appear on the cathode ray tube, input his desired output, and..."poof!"

The Trojan horse perspective is somewhat akin to the iron axe, but with a major difference: the intentions of the Greek gift-bearers were far less benign, and they were far less ignorant about the probable results.

If some among you are wondering what these fairy tales have to do with the urgent and tangible business of improving health in the developing countries, let me present examples of each, transposed into the language of what we choose to call "international health."

I think that the most acute example of the iron axe that I have personally come across was in Iran in the mid-1970s. High ranking Iranian health officials and medical academicians, the large majority of them trained as sub-specialists in the United States, were vying with each other to implant tertiary care facilities all over Tehran. I leave to your imagination the contrast between these efforts and the status of public health services, the availability of primary care, and the access to basic health services for the mass of the population, whether in the mushrooming cities or in the rural areas.

I remember being shown, by a cabinet minister (who was a Boston-trained cardiologist), the plans for a twin tower, 30 story, glass and steel medical complex (designed by a U.S. architectural firm) which was to stand on the edge of Tehran, out towards the airport. One tower was for inpatient services, the other for private physicians' office suites. When I asked the Minister where the outpatient clinics and emergency service were to be located, he replied, "We Iranians don't discriminate as do you Americans between private and ward patients. Everyone will be invited to use the same facility!" I kept to myself any further comment concerning transportation, fees, and other more subtle measures of discrimination, which were at least as prominent in his setting as in my own.

While I do not mean to suggest that the inappropriate modeling of U.S. biomedical technology by elitist Iranian physicians was by itself the iron axe, the story is one that can be repeated about all sectors of the Shah's Iran, complete with multiple groups competing against each other to see who could build the highest tower, abetted by scores of expatriate consultants with briefcases full of plans and samples.

The iron axe of our time is often homegrown in the

developing world.   A few years ago, the Kenyatta National Teaching Hospital in Nairobi, Kenya, was reliably said to consume 75 percent of the health budget of the entire nation!

I remember in my own pediatrics ward on the other coast of Africa, trying to get nurses (Africans trained in the French tradition) to put their support behind efforts to nutritionally rehabilitate the severe kwashiorkor and marasmus patients who formed the bulk of our work. When it came to what was, in essence, regarded as feeding babies, most of the nurses said, "That's not our work, that's for mothers and cooks! We are nurses!"

I would not argue that doctors, nurses, or hospitals are not very important assets in health technology transfer. But will you not agree that there is more than a little iron axe in these, and many hundreds of similar stories?

In contrast, there are, I believe, also some truly magic lamp examples in international health. I have no personal experience with the massive anti-yaws campaigns of the 1950s and early 1960s, but there seems no doubt about the ease, efficiency, and economy of the use of penicillin in community after community.

The eradication of smallpox, which will be discussed later, is another undoubted triumph of the magic lamp.

Two final examples of this positive category: the availability of widespread and effective contraceptive technology, and the development of simple, effective, and economic oral therapy for diarrhea.

All these magic lamp examples have some important characteristics in common. They all represent the application of health technology to a broad mass of population(s), to health problems of major significance, and at application costs that are relatively modest. In most cases, there has been modification of an existing technology developed in the North to meet these reality characteristics of societies in the South. I shall return to this discussion near the end of my paper.

Of course, not all health technologies, even among those that seemed "naturals" for success, have transplanted as well as one might have hoped. For example, the advent of measles vaccine raised high hopes in those of us who have dealt with the devastating impact of this disease among developing country children.   On the surface, the vaccine should have led to effective control, if not near eradication in some communities, of measles.   But the combination of the epidemiology of measles in developing country settings, the logistic problems of heat-unstable vaccine, and the administrative and economic problems of developing country health systems, have led to gains that are far less dramatic than were originally expected.

Another example of somewhat tarnished magic lamps can be seen in the worldwide problems of malaria resurgence, flowing from insecticide resistance of the vector, drug resistance of the parasite, and organizational and delivery problems of the health services.

These examples of only partial success of a highly promising health technology: measles (as an example of lessened effectiveness in the developing country setting) and malaria control (as an example of "second generation" problems--emergence of multiple antibiotic-resistant strains of venereal disease would be another good example of this category) should not be taken as condemnation of the usefulness and benefits of these technologic transfers, but rather of the simple rules that magic lamps are few and far between, and that health workers should be skeptical, prepared for disappointment, quick to anticipate and deal with problems, and resolved to work with even small increments of progress.

Of course, there are many examples of developing country health problems of major importance where our technology does not yet offer even the illusion of a magic lamp, either because of lack of the appropriate technology, or the ability to apply it, or the prohibitive cost of doing so.   Good examples here would be trypanosomiasis, schistosomiasis, and (though it may be surprising to some to see it in this list) leprosy.

Now for the "Trojan horse."   This is a painful and difficult area to speak about in a health context, for the first rule of our profession is "do no harm."   It seems difficult to countenance the possibility that there are any among us who would transfer a health technology while aware of significant harmful effects.

As you may have guessed, the Trojan horse example that I will choose is the aggressive promotion and marketing of infant formula in the Third World.

Hundreds of millions of families in developing countries live in grinding rural poverty or in the urban slums on the septic fringes of modern central cities. I trust that I do not need to acquaint you with the statistics regarding per capita incomes, infant mortality rates, life expectancies, illiteracy, etc., that distinguish these populations from those of the more affluent countries. But these two great divisions among mankind--the poor and the rich (within, as well as between the South and the North) are no longer separated by space and time as were the Australian tribe and the European anthropologists. These two great cultures of mankind no longer come <u>episodically</u> into, to use Alan Morehead's phrase, "fatal impact." Rich and poor, North and South, "developed" and "less developed," modern and traditional, are now interpenetrated both in space and time, continuously influencing each other. What happens when the technologic achievements of the North, designed, developed, and often controlled in and by the industrially affluent culture, without initial thought for the implications for the other culture of humankind, flow across cultural and national frontiers?

In all settings, both in affluent and developing nations, breast feeding of infants is superior to bottle feeding. Breast milk contains antibodies which protect the infant against infectious disease; breast milk is never allergenic; breast feeding offers a natural family planning and child-spacing mechanism because of lactation's inhibition of ovulation; breast feeding is a very important aid to positive psycho-social bonding between mother and infant. Breast milk is not contaminated by polluted water, nor by flies and other insects, and breast milk is a naturally tested and evolutionarily proven food. There is no serious argument against these many advantages of breast versus bottle feeding.

In the developing countries where poverty is the rule of life, where polluted water sources are ubiquitous, where health services are few and far between, where the majority of mothers are illiterate, where a wide range of infectious and parasitic diseases threaten mothers and children--in these settings the baby bottle can be a lethal weapon--highly likely to be contaminated, often filled with over diluted formula by an unsuspecting mother trying to stretch a meager family budget.

Almost 100 million infants are born in the developing world each year. One in 10 of these infants does not live to see their first birthday--that comes to 10 million infant deaths annually in the developing world. Half of these deaths (about 5 million annually) are due to the vicious cycle of diarrhea and malnutrition. Of these 5 million deaths, the best available estimates are that up to 1 million deaths are directly attributable to the association of contaminated infant formula with diarrhea and malnutrition. These estimates are based on World Health Organization and UNICEF projections, upon estimates drawn from studies in local areas, and upon the field experience of hundreds of health professionals. This well known association led to the coining of the term, almost a decade ago, of "commerciogenic malnutrition"--its existence and its prevalence is as well known to health workers in developing countries as is malaria or trachoma.

In the settings that I am describing, the advertising and mass marketing practices of the infant formula manufacturers reinforce, accentuate, and even create, patterns of cultural change that lead to rapid declines of breast feeding among mothers living in poverty.

Dr. David Morley is the pediatrician who introduced the concept of health care aimed at the "under-fives." In his 1973 textbook, Pediatric Priorities in the Developing World, Morley says, "In many countries, artificial feeding has come to stay, not only in the large cities amongst the wealthier members of the population, but also in rural areas. This is largely due to a belief in the 'prestige' of artificial milk developed by the manufacturers of artificial foods determined to sell their particular brand." 1/

Dr. Cicely Williams is the pioneer of international child nutrition. It was she who in 1933 first described protein-calorie malnutrition, "kwashiorkor," while working in West Africa. In 1972 in Maternal and Child Health: Delivering the Services, she says along with her co-author:

> "Most significantly, a falling-off of breast feeding is usually found, partly because some mothers may have to work in town in employment where breast feeding is taboo by modern convention, but also because of the unfortunate imitation of the apparently statusful bottle feeding carried out by socioeconomic superiors, and because of harmful effects of ill-advised and inappropriate advertis-

ing of expensive proprietary milk preparations, and because of widespread lack of knowledge of breast feeding on the part of health staff...Fifteen years ago, 'bottle feeding disease' was uncommon in Mulago Hospital, Kampala; by the mid-1960s, it accounted for 10-15 percent of pediatric admissions." 2/

Professor Derrick Jelliffe chairs the Department of Maternal and Child Health and International Health at UCLA School of Public Health; he is the world's foremost authority on the interactions of tropical child health and nutrition and the author/editor of the standard textbook of diseases of children in the tropics and subtropics. In the 1978 text which he and his wife co-authored, Human Milk in the Modern World, they say:

"To compensate for declining sales in the U.S.A. and Europe, an increasing drive has developed for sales overseas in resource-poor countries, where marketing surveillance is negligible and large populations using small quantities could still add substantial sales. By creating a need, sales can be expanded down the income ladder. Techniques employed in sales promotion include 'milk nurses', 'formula banks', free samples to mothers and to health services, widespread distribution of 'educational' promotional material, prizes, contests, lotteries, contrived news items, displays at 'point of purchase' and on labels, and assistance to health professionals, as well as advertising through the mass media." 3/

In his clinical textbook, Jelliffe states that:

"The dangers of artificial feeding in the average tropical home cannot be overstressed and, in many lower socioeconomic circumstances, chances of success are slight. The result is only too likely to be a development of nutritional marasmus from over-diluted mixtures, and associated infective diarrhea from the use of contaminated feeds given in unclean utensils." 4/

No one disputes the value of the technologic advance of the development of standardized and nutritious commercial infant formula in the United States and Europe since about

1930, in settings where mothers were massively abandoning breast feeding <u>and</u> where economic and hygienic circumstances were such as to minimize the dangers of artificial feeding. I must say, parenthetically, that there is recent evidence that formula feeding in the United States may not be so benign as was once thought 5/, but the hazards are certainly of a lesser order of magnitude than in the Third World.

Infant formula was developed for marketing in affluent societies. The vast potential of untapped developing countries markets soon attracted the attention of the industry. No one disputes that there is a role for infant formula in developing countries; the issue is what role, under what conditions of appropriateness.

As the global debate over the World Health Organization's infant marketing code demonstrated 6/, 7/, the mass marketing and high pressure promotion of infant formula to poverty populations in developing countries is not an acceptable technology transfer, from either health or economic perspectives. Those who engage in these practices are either closing their eyes to the consequences of their actions, or deliberately exporting a Trojan horse.

Unfortunately, the infant formula issue is not the sole example of contemporary Trojan horses. The dumping of outdated pharmaceutical products, the export of banned or severely restricted pesticides and herbicides, double standards regarding toxicity and limitations-of-use warnings on drugs manufactured by the same company but sold in multiple countries--these and other examples fall in the same category. As the health and agricultural technologies generated by recombinant DNA research come onstream over the next very few years, we will find ourselves, as a global species, needing to pay major attention to the Trojan horse issue. We do not currently have adequate institutions and mechanisms to deal with these cross-cultural and transnational problems.

The preceding examples of all three perspective categories--iron axe, magic lamp, and Trojan horse--have urgent importance, not only in their own right as we ponder the transfer of biomedical technology from North to South, but also as case examples of even larger questions that go far beyond the health sector.

Humankind, as a species, is now faced with a series of

major issues that have the following characteristice in common:

(a) They are global in nature. No longer do the anthropologists descend on the aborigines out of the blue--each
and every part of the of the globe today has direct and significant interaction--and impact--on each and every other
part.

(b) They (these major issues) are highly technologically complex in nature. Whether we are talking about acid
rain, greenhouse effect, nuclear power, or multiple species
extinction because of rain forest destruction--there are no
simple equations or unilateral relationships.

(c) These issues involve economic and/or political
conflict across cultural and national frontiers.

These issues, as you can deduce from all the examples I
have presented, often appear in the guise of health and/or
nutrition problems, though they are actually of much larger
dimension, involving the deepest questions concerning who we
recognize as "us" and who as "them," and what our responsibilities are to "us" and "them."

To return to the level of discussion concerning the
transfer of health technology between North and South, an
analogy is often drawn between the demographic/disease
patterns of today's developing countries and those of Europe
and North America a century or more ago. It is true that
the combination of high birth rates, high death rates, and
high levels of morbidity and mortality based on infectious
disease, malnutrition, polluted water, and mass poverty
could describe either setting.

Are any of you familiar with the source of the following passage?

"'Protect us, O God, from diphtheria!' These
ringing words uttered by my father at morning
prayers were my first introduction to the tragedy
of diseases. The atmosphere in our home that
morning was tense...Some hours later a long line
of teams came slowly down that road. Driving the
lead team, a strange one, was my father, and be-
side him sat a man I did not know. In the bed of
the farm wagon were three oblong boxes. Following
were spring wagons, farm wagons, and a large

number of men on horseback. Questions directed to my mother brought no answer. Father returned home after many hours and cryptically announced as he came in the door: 'Five more.'

"As days wore on I learned that the wagon had borne the coffins containing the bodies of three of my playmates. Five more followed in quick succession. Eight of the nine children in that one family died of diphtheria in ten days. There remained only a baby of nine months. The mother took to carrying this child constantly even while she did the farm housework..."

Indeed, there is a close analogy between the developing world of today and the life setting of our entire species just a short while ago. The above passage was not written by a Latin American physician, nor by a medical missionary in contemporary India. It was written by Dr. Arthur E. Hertzler, in 1938, recalling his boyhood on the Kansas frontier after the Civil War. 8/ Life was hard in western Kansas, less than 150 years ago. Perhaps the same level of protein-energy malnutrition, polluted water, and the worst effects of mass poverty as are found today in the Third World were not present, but the common communicable childhood disease patterns were quite similar. In the crowded cities of 18th and 19th century Europe and North America, conditions were even more similar to the Bombays and the Bogotas of today.

There is another important lesson to be found in Dr. Hertzler's book, The Horse and Buggy Doctor. Written in 1938, the state of the medical art had moved light years from that obtained during his boyhood. By 1938, Dr. Hertzler was not only in posession of diphtheria vaccine and antitoxin, but there were also many doctors, and many hospitals, in western Kansas. Sulfa drugs were just coming in, and the magic lamp of penicillin was less than a decade away. Surgical and anesthetic techniques had been revolutionized.

Of course, if we compare the technology of today, 1981, with that of 1938, it reveals an even greater quantum leap than between 1870 and 1938. And how will 2008 compare to 1981?

The point is, of course, that one enormous difference between the developing countries today and the health situation in Kansas or New York City a century or so ago is that today humankind is in posession of a biomedical technology that, for all its problems, exists, is highly effective for many major problems, and is available for transfer for the benefit of all, requiring only that we (and by we, I mean all of us, in developing as well as affluent countries) figure out how to apply that technology appropriately, equitably, and at an affordable cost.

Granted, it is the broad socioeconomic condition of a society that is the primary determinant of its level of health and the shape of its disease pattern. The biomedical technology is not going to eradicate global protein-energy malnutrition. The more than 50 percent of our species who lack access to clean drinking water do not suffer that lack principally because of a failure of the biomedical technology. But this line of argument is too often overstated. There are enormous improvements in the world's health that can be achieved by application of existing and soon-to-come technology. We should be cautioned by the iron axe, do battle against the Trojan horse, but work with even the brass reproductions of the magic lamp.

In 1978, at Alma Ata, the world health community of nations accepted the challenge of providing "Health for All by the Year 2000." This slogan is often criticized as being utopian and unachievable. By "Health for All," however, the World Health Organization (WHO) does not mean the absence of disease, nor even the control of major epidemic and endemic maladies, but rather, in the words of WHO's Director General, Halfdan Mahler, "Access to some basic, decent level of health care for all individuals." I, for one, believe this latter goal is possible to achieve, that sufficient resources, financial and human, can be mobilized over the next 20 years, if we have the collective will to do so. 9/

Whether or not you agree with me as to feasibility, I trust that you will agree that the major barriers to "Health for All" do not lie in the absence of technologic fixes, nor that substantial progress could only occur after our biomedical knowledge is increased by some quantum amount.

The major "Health for All" barriers are economic and political, and involve obstacles to the application of existing technology. This should not be taken as an argument against the need for continued research. Laboratory, clinical, epidemiological, and health services research are continuously required, to improve efficiency and effectiveness, and to overcome the many significant biomedical problems for which no satisfactory technologic solution currently exists (for example, schistomiasis).

But, if we could bend a major portion of our efforts in this business of the transfer of health technology towards a better understanding of how to transfer by technologically appropriate means (as regards level of technologic sophistication, carrying capacity of administrative and logistic systems, and financial and human resource availability) with widespread and equitable distribution of results, we would take the longest and most important step possible in the pursuit of "Health for All."

What an incredible achievement is represented by the global eradication of smallpox! I lived and worked in Nepal in the early 1960s; if I had been told that smallpox would disappear, forever, among those mountain valleys within 15 years, I would not have believed it. Yet, it was done. Smallpox eradication is the brightest example, in my view, of the magic lamp of the transfer of health technology on a global basis. It benefitted every human being; it was done at an annual cost far less than the annual cost of smallpox prevention, diagnosis, and treatment; and it represented a cooperative effort not only between North and South, but between all nations.

Let us look at the key elements that made this success possible. First, there is the matter of technologic advance. There were two main recent breakthroughs leading to smallpox eradication. One was rather sophisticated--development of an improved freeze-dried vaccine. The other was a marvelous example of unsophisticated low-cost technology--the development of the bifurcated needle, hardly a space age stride. It displaced the expensive and trouble-prone jet injector and the old single-prong needle. In its simplicity lay its appropriateness.

The second major factor in the eradication of smallpox was the administrative and managerial skill brought to the campaign. Epidemiologic and health services research were brilliantly combined with applied principles of the management, behavioral, and political sciences.

The third, and in my view the most important factor was the genuinely global cooperation between nations (note I said "genuine" and not "trouble free"). Not only was the spirit of the smallpox eradication campaign truly international--it rose above a perspective of "from the developed to the developing" to one of "among countries for our mutual benefit." If these words sound naive in these cynical times, I ask anyone to provide an alternative description of the history.

Just as the eradication of smallpox provides an example of how effective and productive the international transfer of health technology can be, so the infant formula marketing controversy provides an example of the worst end of the spectrum; an expensive technology for which over 90 percent of women have no biologic need, for which a mass market is created rather than responded to, a transfer that involves great hazards to the health and life of children when this technology is transferred to the economic, sanitary, and morbidity context of developing countries, a technologic transfer that benefits few and injures many.

Neither the eradication of smallpox nor the sale of infant formula will determine the biologic survival of our species. Neither issue would show up very high on any really "macro" list of transfer of technology issues. The greatest importance of both of them lies in the examples that they set for the ways in which we can, by our own choices, cope with cross-cultural and transnational transfer issues: iron axe, Trojan horse, or magic lamp.

The author's current research is supported in part by a grant from the International Development Research Center of Canada. The author is solely responsible for all opinions expressed in this article.

Footnotes

1. Morley, D. Pediatric Priorities in the Developing World. Butterworths, 1973, page 118.

2. Williams, C.D. and Jelliffe, D.B. Maternal and Child Health: Delivering the Services. London: Oxford University Press, 1972, page 9.

3. Jelliffe, D.B. and Jelliffe, E.F. Human Milk in the Modern World. New York, NY: Oxford University Press, 1978, page 340.

4. Jelliffe, D.B. and Stanfield, J.P. (eds). Diseases of Children in the Subtropics and Tropics. London: Edward Arnold Publishers, 1978, 3rd Ed., page 176.

5. Cunningham, A.S. "Breast-feeding and Morbidity in Industrialized Countries: an Update." Advances in International Maternal and Child Health: Volume 1, edited by D.B. and E.F.P. Jelliffe. New York, NY: Oxford University Press, 1982, pages 128-169.

6. Joseph, S.C. "The Anatomy of the Infant Formula Controvery." American Journal of Diseases of Children. Vol. 135 (October 1981), pages 889-892.

7. Graham, G.G. "Comments on the World Health Organization 'International Code' of Breast Milk Substitutes." American Journal of Disease of Children. Vol. 135 (October 1981), pages 892-894.

8. Hertzler, A.E. The Horse and Buggy Doctor. Lincoln, NB: University of Nebraska Press, 1970, page 1.

9. Joseph, S.C. and Russell, S.S. "Is Primary Care the Wave of the Future?" Social Science and Medicine. Vol. 14c (1980), pages 137-144.

ECONOMIC IMPACT AND COST-EFFECTIVENESS OF MEDICAL TECHNOLOGY
Milton C. Weinstein, Ph.D.

A major contributor to the rising costs of health care in the United States has been the increasing use of medical technology. Costs of equipment, of procedures made possible or more frequent by new technology, and of procedures induced by the diagnostic information or therapeutic consequences of technology, all contribute.

Cost-effectiveness analysis has been proposed as a method by which to evaluate the health benefits of a technology in relation to its net economic impact, so that priorities for the use of limited resources can be set. Cost-effectiveness analysis may be of value to policymakers, fiscal intermediaries, health care institutions, and clinicians, although current institutional incentives do not favor its rapid dissemination.

Recent applications of cost-effectiveness analysis to interventions in cardiovascular disease suggest that coronary artery bypass surgery for multiple vessels, coronary angiography in definite angina, and treatment of moderate to severe diastolic hypertension are all relatively cost-effective, while screening for coronary disease using radionuclide scanning or angiography, and treatment of borderline hypertension are substantially less cost-effective. Coronary artery bypass surgery for single vessel disease, screening of asymptomatic adult males with exercise stress testing, screening for hypertension, and treatment of mild hypertension are intermediate in their cost-effectiveness.

Limitations of cost-effectiveness evaluations include their reliance on subjective estimates of uncertain effects of treatment, their sensitivity to value judgments concerning health outcomes, and the danger that other social values such as interpersonal equity, or psychological factors such as the patient's anxiety, may be ignored.   Nonetheless, such economic evaluations should complement evaluations of clinical efficacy in guiding the use of medical resources by providers and policymakers.

Medical Technology and the Rise in Health Care Costs

In 1981, the United States will have spent over $260 billion on health care (Freeland et al., 1980).   During the 1970s, expenditures on health care tripled, increasing at double-digit rates in every year, and averaging 14.7 percent per year.   Meanwhile, the consumer price index was increasing by less than half that rate (U.S. Department of Health and Human Services, 1980). It might be suspected that population increases, or shifts in the age distribution toward the elderly, might account for these trends; however, a study which adjusted for inflation, age mix, and population size found that the real, age-adjusted, per capita expenditure on health care rose by 4.5 percent per year. As a fraction of the gross national product (GNP), health care's share has increased steadily, from 3.5 percent in 1929, to 5.3 percent in 1960, to 7.6 percent in 1970, to more than 9 percent in 1980 (U.S. Department of Health and Human Services, 1980).

A much analyzed question is to what degree technology has contributed to the increase in medical care costs (Banta et al., 1981).   To begin to address this question, one needs a definition of medical technology, and I shall adopt the one proposed by the Office of Technology Assessment:

> "The drugs, devices, and medical and surgical procedures used in medical care, and the organizational and supportive systems within which such care is provided."   (Office of Technology Assessment, 1978a).

New technology, then, includes but is not limited to new drugs, new procedures--either equipment-embodied (such as computed tomography) or not (such as coronary artery bypass surgery)--and new modes of delivery (such as neonatal and coronary intensive care units).   Much of the research to which I have referred has concentrated on hospital costs, and is based on the premise that increases in price-adjusted costs per hospital day may be attributed, by default, to technology.   Thus, of the average annual increase of 14.7

percent in hospital costs during 1970-1979, 8.2 percent could be explained by price increases (for wages, supplies, utilities, etc.), and only 1.7 percent by increased utilization (that is, bed days), leaving 4.2 percent, or about 30 percent of the total and 70 percent of the price-adjusted total, unexplained and presumably attributable to technology (U.S. Department of Health and Human Services, 1980). A study for the Council on Wage and Price Stability reached a similar conclusion that about 75 percent of the increases in price-adjusted costs could be attributable to technology (Feldstein and Taylor, 1977).

Whether or not technology is the "culprit behind health care costs," as the question was posed in a 1977 conference on the topic (Altman and Blendon, 1979), there is ample evidence that the use of certain technologies has been rapidly increasing. The number of coronary artery bypass operations, for example, has grown from virtually zero a decade ago to an estimated 110,000 in 1980, and now consumes more expenditures than any other surgical operation. Combined with coronary arteriography, it accounts for more than one percent of all health care expenditures. Not only expensive, high visibility procedures, however, are responsible for all of the cost increases. Laboratory tests, while inexpensive on a unit basis, have grown in volume to such an extent that their share of the cost of a hospital day has increased despite a decrease in the cost per test performed (Scitovsky and McCall, 1976; Fineberg, 1979). It must be observed, however, that some technologies may actually decrease costs, by substituting for physician services, obviating hospital admissions or reducing length of stay, or preventing later occurrence of illness.

There are many processes by which technologies can affect health care costs. The first, and most direct, pertains to capital-intensive, equipment-embodied technologies, for which the cost of the equipment itself is sufficient to give cause for concern. Certificate-of-need laws have attempted to control this component of technology induced costs. Computed tomography and coronary intensive care units are prime examples.

A second mechanism by which a technology affects costs is by means of its impact on operating costs. Surgical procedures, and other procedures that require highly skilled professional labor, would be of this type. However, studies have estimated that even equipment-embodied technologies can have their greatest economic impact on operating costs. For

example, for computed cranial tomography, it has been estimated that 50 to 75 percent of the cost of performing head
scans in a reasonably well-utilized unit are attributable to
operating and maintaining the equipment, as distinguished
from capital costs (Office of Technology Assessment, 1978b).

A third, and even less direct, sort of impact on costs
is exemplified by automation in the clinical laboratory, and
concerns the ability of a technology to facilitate performing a service at very high volumes. A decrease in unit
costs, or time, may induce increased utilization to a point
beyond that at which the procedures are cost-effective, or
even beneficial (Weinstein and Pearlman, 1981).

The fourth process by which technologies can lead to
higher costs, and most difficult to foresee, is by affecting
the use of additional procedures which are themselves
costly. For example, electronic fetal monitoring is not an
extraordinarily costly procedure, but if its use results in
an increased rate of Cesarean section deliveries, then the
induced costs of surgery--which have been estimated to be
nearly three times as great as those of monitoring itself
(Banta and Thacker, 1979)--would be the major health care
cost attributable to the technology. Technologies can also
have cost-reducing effects, by obviating the use of other
procedures. This might be expected if a new technology
supplants--rather than augments--an existing one, or if a
preventive technology is effective at reducing the incidence
of disease.

The Need for Cost-Effectiveness Evaluation

I will not attempt to review the many forces--economic,
sociologic, behavioral, political, and ethical--that drive
the use of medical technology, especially new technology.
Undoubtedly, for some physicians, the profit motive plays a
role. Other factors, including the provider's and patient's
mutual desire for the best, most modern health care available, also are involved.

Whatever the forces, medical practice is filled with
technologies whose efficacy has not been adequately tested,
and whose impact on cost could be great. Some of these,
like the practice of gastric freezing during the 1960s, are
not efficacious and may consume millions or even billions of
health care dollars before they are abandoned. Others offer
benefits to some patients, but perhaps at a cost that raises
the question of whether one can afford to spend unlimited

resources to achieve every possible health benefit.   Still others are truly cost-effective; they provide valuable bene- fits at a reasonable cost.   For each new procedure that comes along, we should ask where along this continuum it lies, or is likely to lie.

Given the limited resources available, the question is not whether a million dollars, or 10 million dollars, or 100 million dollars is more than a life is worth, but whether we are allocating our resources among the competing available uses and technologies, in the manner that will provide the greatest possible health benefit for the society.   While evaluations of efficacy, such as clinical trials, can be counted on to identify some technologies that are truly inefficacious, clinical trials cannot be counted on, even in the long run, to eliminate the need for difficult choices among those competing uses of health care resources that may offer some benefits, given the unavoidable uncertainties in medical decision making.   Thus, evaluation of medical tech- nology must go beyond evaluation of efficacy, and must con- sider the relation between efficacy--or, more properly, effectiveness in actual medical practice--and health care resource cost.   This is the objective of cost-effectiveness analysis.

Principles of Cost-Effectiveness Analysis

The purpose of cost-effectiveness analysis, then, is to assess the efficiency with which limited resources are being allocated to achieve the desired benefits.   The implicit assumption is that the objective is to maximize the aggre- gate health benefits, or effectiveness, obtainable from a given level of expenditures, or cost.   This approach leads to the use of a cost-effectiveness ratio--net resource cost per unit of net effectiveness--as a yardstick for ranking alternative uses of resources.

1.   Perspective

The findings of cost-effectiveness analysis may be use- ful in decision making not only for populations of patients but also for individual patients, provided that the latter decisions are faced in the context of explicitly limited resources or incentives to control costs.   Because of the conflicting objectives of various parties to decision making, an analysis is most useful if it makes explicit its perspective, be it that of the individual patient, a hospital, a government agency, a health maintenance organization, or the society at large.

2.   Costs

Assuming the societal perspective, it has become customary to define "cost" as the net health care resource cost, that is, the net burden on the health care budget. For a treatment, net resource cost includes the cost of treatment itself, including follow-up treatments and tests to monitor the course of therapy; the costs of treating side effects and complications of treatment; and the savings resulting from the prevention of subsequent morbidity. For a diagnostic test, one must include the testing costs, as well as the induced costs and savings for tests and treatments added or averted as a result of the diagnostic information. The example of noninvasive tests for coronary artery disease illustrates this point about induced costs and savings. In symptomatic patients, performing an exercise stress test can obviate angiography and its costs in many patients who test negative, while in asymptomatic patients, a positive stress test can lead to angiography and, perhaps, surgery in patients who would not otherwise receive them.

Ideally, in an analysis from the societal perspective, costs should be measured as the value of real resources actually consumed, irrespective of the amount of money that changes hands as reimbursement. Data on true costs of particular procedures are rare, however, and costly to obtain. Hence, the analyst is usually forced to rely on charges as proxies for costs, despite the errors introduced.

3.   Effectiveness

Health effectiveness may be measured in any of several units, the only requirement in a cost-effectiveness analysis being that a single measure be used so that alternative uses of resources may be compared. Occasionally an intermediate measure, short of a final health outcome, is used, such as the number of cases of disease found by a diagnostic test. It is more desireable, though, to measure health effectiveness in units more transferable across technologies, such as the number of years of life saved.

But longevity may not be the only outcome of importance; effects on the quality of life, including symptoms and functional status, may be of concern. Trade-offs among health states, and between longevity and quality of life, may be involved. Effects due to side effects of treatments, morbidity averted, and symptom relief, must all be considered.

One class of methods for valuing outcomes in cost-effectiveness studies is to assign weights (on a 0-1 scale) to time spent in various health states, to yield quality-adjusted life expectancy as the measure of effectiveness. (Kaplan et al., 1976; Torrance, 1976; Weinstein and Stason, 1977).

For example, in coronary bypass surgery, a pivotal issue is the degree to which a patient would be willing to give up life expectancy for relief from angina pectoris. The time-tradeoff (Figure 1) approach seeks a balance between some number of years with angina and some fraction, Q, of that number of years that a patient would accept to be free of angina. For example, a patient might be willing to trade 10 years with his severe angina for 7 years without angina. For this patient, one year at his level of angina would be worth 0.7 quality-adjusted life years (QALY). For a patient with milder angina or a more sedentary lifestyle, the weight assigned to one year with angina would be higher, say 0.9. For a patient with extremely severe angina or extreme psychological problems owing to the angina, a weight of 0.5, reflecting a willingness to give up half his remaining life span to be rid of the angina, might be plausible.

Inevitably, the more comprehensive a measure of benefit is desired, the more value judgments enter into the analysis in the process of commensurating diverse outcomes. However, to omit quality of life and other "intangible" considerations because of difficulties in measurement would be irresponsible if those considerations are central to the concerns of the physician, the patient, or the society at large.

4.   Interpreting the Cost-Effectiveness Ratio

When based on suitable measures of resource cost and of health effectiveness, the ratio of cost per unit of effectiveness (for example, dollars per quality-adjusted year of life gained) provides a yardstick that can be used to guide the setting of priorities for resource allocation. Given a budget, and given cost-effectiveness ratios for a variety of technologies in various uses, the way to achieve the maximum benefit would be to rank the alternative expenditures from the lowest value of the ratio to the highest, and to select in order of priority until either the budget is exhausted or society determines somehow that the next dollar of expenditure is not justified by the benefits. Procedures would be adopted down as far as the cut-off point, where the choice of the cut-off point, whether it were $50,000 or $1 million, per QALY, could be determined by the availability of resources.

5.   Discounting the Future

A problem arises, with respect to the weighing of costs and health effects that occur at different points in time. This process is usually accomplished in two steps: (1) adjusting all costs for inflation; and (2) discounting future costs and health effects at an appropriate interest rate, usually between 5 and 10 percent per year after inflation.

The practice of discounting future costs is not controversial; the same cannot be said of discounting future health risks and benefits. The argument for discounting says that failure to discount implies inefficiency in the use of medical resources: Why spend today's resources to buy future health if we could invest those resources and have more resources available to buy even more health at that time in the future? (Weinstein and Stason, 1977).

6.   Equity

Another value issue concerns the aggregation of costs and benefits into a single number regardless of who pays the bill or who receives the benefits. Many analysts cope with the equity problem by ignoring it; this practice is clearly inappropriate in principle. At a minimum, the policy analyst should examine whether the distribution of costs and benefits appears to be socially desirable (e.g., by redistributing welfare from the rich to the poor, or from those who lead a healthy lifestyle to those who do not).

Cost-Effectiveness Analysis and Cardiovascular Disease

To illustrate the kinds of insights that can be drawn from cost-effectiveness analysis, the results of several studies that my colleagues and I have conducted in the domain of cardiovascular disease are summarized. The technologies evaluated represent the range of clinical interventions, from treatment, to diagnosis, to screening, to prevention. Treatment is exemplified by coronary artery bypass surgery (CABS), diagnosis by the use of coronary angiography in symptomatic patients, screening by the use of radionuclide scanning and exercise tolerance testing in asymptomatic persons, and prevention by the detection and management of hypertension. Results from these analyses can be applied at several levels. They can be useful in guiding priorities within each of these classes of intervention into the disease (e.g., What patients should get the highest priority for antihypertensive treatment or for coronary artery bypass surgery? What is the most cost effective strategy for detecting hypertensives or for diagnosing coronary artery disease?). Taking the results a step further and comparing cost-effectiveness of prevention versus screening versus diagnosis versus treatment can yield insights at the higher level of allocating resources among these broad classes of interventions into the disease. Or, one can go even further and compare interventions in coronary artery disease with those for diagnosis and treatment of cancer, or ulcer disease, or gynecologic disorders. It is to be hoped that the proliferation of cost-effectiveness studies over a broad range of technologies and diseases will make such comparisons possible.

1.   Coronary Artery Bypass Surgery (CABS)
     (Weinstein and Stason, in press)

Methods. Our analysis of CABS applies to a population of 55-year-old males with operable coronary artery disease, 50 percent or more arterial obstruction, and good ventricular function.

Mortality rates were obtained from the European Coronary Surgery Study, the Veterans Administration (VA) trial, and two large data banks.

To incorporate quality of life considerations, including both physical and psychological factors, we selected a spectrum of preference weights for the present level of angina, ranging from Q=1, representing concern for life years alone, to Q=0.5 for extremely severe angina. Our central assumption is a value of Q=0.7, reflecting moderately severe angina and a preference for an active lifestyle.

Net resource costs of CABS consist of: (1) the cost of surgery itself, estimated at between $15,000 and $20,000 in 1981; (2) savings in medical management costs; and (3) savings owing to the prevention of myocardial infarctions.

All future costs and benefits were discounted to present value, at five percent per year.

Results. Under our central assumptions, surgery results in a small loss of life expectancy (0.2 years) for one-
vessel disease, a gain of 0.6 years for two-vessel disease and
gains of 3.2 and 6.9 years for three-vessel and left-main
disease, respectively. Using the higher operative mortality
rates derived from the VA study reduced the estimated benefits of surgery, but in no case did medical management become superior.

Figure 2 shows the differences in quality-adjusted life
expectancy, as a function of the severity, or perceived
severity, of angina as reflected in the quality weights.
Using a weight of 0.7 for the present (severe) level of
angina, surgery is seen to be preferable even for one-vessel
disease when symptom relief is taken into account.

The expected net resource cost of surgical treatment
was estimated to be $14,000 for patients with severe angina,
and $15,500 for patients with mild angina. The net cost for
mild angina is higher than for severe angina because the
amount of medication costs averted is smaller than with
severe angina.

These estimates of net resource costs and health effectiveness provide the basis for estimating the cost-effectiveness of CABS. Recall that the lower the value of the
ratio of net resource cost to gain in quality-adjusted life
expectancy, the more attractive surgery is as a use of medical resources.

For patients with severe angina, the cost per year of
quality-adjusted life expectancy gained ranges from $3,800
for left-main disease to $30,000 for one-vessel disease
(Figure 3). Two-vessel and three-vessel disease are intermediate at $17,500 to $7,200 respectively. While it is
difficult to interpret these figures in isolation, it will
be shown subsequently that they compare favorably with
those for the treatment of essential hypertension.

A sensitivity analysis with respect to the perceived
severity of angina is shown in Figure 4.

For one-vessel disease, and ignoring symptom relief
(Q=1.0), the net effectiveness is negative, so the cost-
effectiveness ratio is undefined. When angina is perceived
as mild (Q=0.9), the cost per quality adjusted year gained

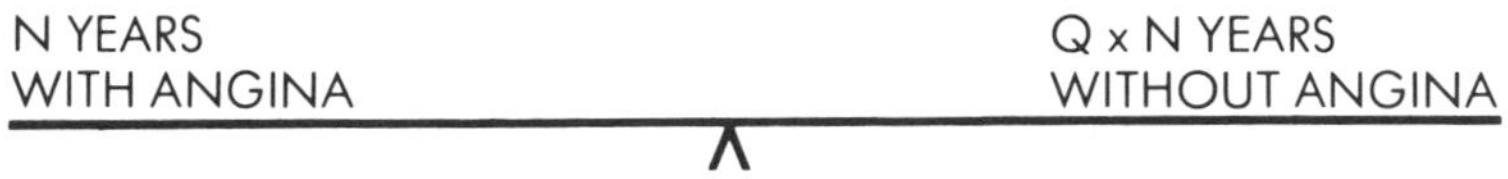

N YEARS
WITH ANGINA

Q x N YEARS
WITHOUT ANGINA

Figure 1. Schematic representation of the time-tradeoff approach to quality-of-life adjustment. (Source: Weinstein and Stason, in press)

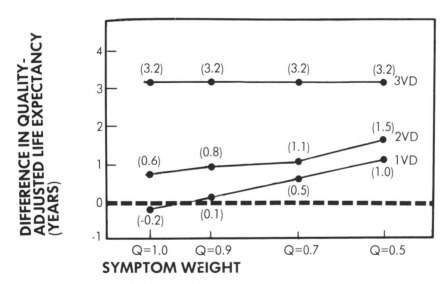

Figure 2. Estimated differences in quality-adjusted life expectancy between surgery and medical management, by number of diseased vessels and quality weights.

Q = 1.0 is equivalent to no angina or no concern over pain;
Q = 0.9 is equivalent to mild angina and a sedentary life style;
Q = 0.7 is equivalent to severe angina and an active life style;
Q = 0.5 is equivalent to very severe angina or serious psychological effects.
(Source: Weinstein and Stason, in press)

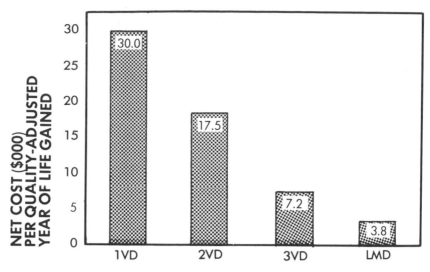

Figure 3. Cost-effectiveness of coronary artery bypass surgery, by number of diseased vessels.
(Central assumptions, severe angina (Q=0.7), present values at 5% per annum.)

1VD=one-vessel disease; 2VD=two-vessel disease;
3VD=three-vessel disease; LMD=left-main disease.
(Source: Weinstein and Stason, in press)

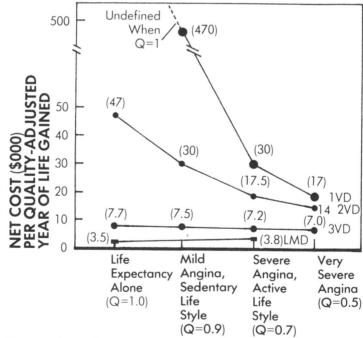

Figure 4. Cost-effectiveness of coronary artery bypass surgery, as a function of the perceived severity of angina

(Central assumptions; present values at 5% per annum.)
1VD=one-vessel disease; 2VD=two-vessel disease; 3VD=three-vessel disease; LMD=left-main disease.
(Source: Weinstein and Stason, in press)

is $470,000. When the angina is perceived as severe (Q=0.7) or very severe (Q=0.5), however, the cost-effectiveness ratios fall to $30,000 and $17,000 per quality-adjusted year, respectively. Thus, for one-vessel disease, the value attached to symptom relief is critical.

For two-vessel disease, the effect of symptom relief remains important, as the cost-effectiveness ratio falls from $47,000 per year of life gained if quality of life is ignored (Q=1) to $14,000 per quality-adjusted year gained if angina is perceived to be very severe (Q=0.5).

In three-vessel and left-main disease, the symptom relief is dominated by the effects on survival, so the cost-effectiveness ratio varies only slightly as the perceived disutility of angina is varied.

2.   Coronary Angiography in Diagnosis
     (Weinstein and Stason, in press)

Having evaluated the cost effectiveness of CABS, let us now step back to the prior stage of diagnosis of coronary disease in a population with anginal symptoms. The cost effectiveness of coronary angiography depends on the costs and risks of angiography, on its yields of valid diagnostic information, and on the cost-effectiveness of subsequent treatment by surgery.

Methods. The cost of angiography was estimated to be about $2,000. The yield of angiography in symptomatic patients was estimated, from various sources, to be about four bypass operations for every 10 angiograms performed. Mortality from angiography is between one and two per thousand.

Results. Cost-effectiveness ratios were calculated for three cases (Figure 5), reflecting a range of operative mortality rates and costs, and varying weights attached to symptom relief.

In the central case, the net cost per quality-adjusted year of life gained is $15,500 overall, $14,000 if patients with one-vessel disease are excluded from surgery, and $12,500 if patients with two-vessel disease are also excluded.

3.   Screening for Coronary Artery Disease
     (Fineberg and Stason, in press)

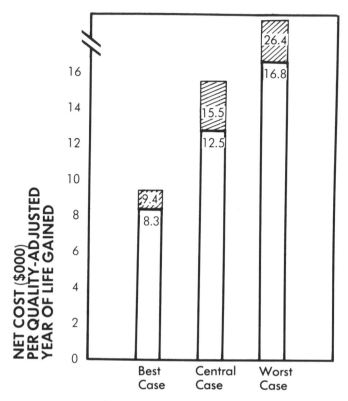

Figure 5. Cost-effectiveness of coronary angiography.
Best Case: Extrapolated mortality assumption, low net cost assumptions, severe angina (Q=0.7).

Central Case: Central mortality assumption, central net cost assumptions, severe angina (Q=0.7).

Worst Case: High operative mortality assumption, high net cost assumptions, symptoms ignored (Q=1.0).

Within each case, the upper figure assumes that all patients with operable disease are given surgery; the lower figure in the best case excludes one-vessel disease from surgery and in the central and worst cases excludes one- and two-vessel disease from surgery to optimize the use of resources.

(Source: Weinstein and Stason, in press)

Screening has been a favored activity among those who advocated preventive medicine. A surge of enthusiasm for radionuclide scanning (RNS), exercise tolerance testing (ETT), and even coronary angiography as primary screening tests in asymptomatic patients, has been evident recently, especially in the light of the successes of coronary artery surgery.

Methods. Fineberg and Stason evaluated five strategies for screening asymptomatic patients (Table 1): (1) angiography as a primary screen; (2) RNS, followed by angiography if positive; (3) ETT, followed by angiography if positive; (4) RNS, followed by ETT if positive, followed by angiography if both positive; and (5) ETT, followed by RNS if positive, followed by angiography if both positive. In all cases, it was assumed that surgery would be performed in operable multiple-vessel disease, which was estimated to occur in 2.5 percent of asymptomatic male patients, averaging 55 years of age. Data on the diagnostic accuracy of the tests were obtained from several clinical studies, and costs were estimated from local hospital charges. Effects of surgery on life expectancy were based on the analysis just presented (Weinstein and Stason, in press). Benefits were discounted to present value at an annual rate of five percent.

Results. Analysis of results in terms of incremental costs and benefits as one progresses to increasingly costly, yet more beneficial, strategies is instructive (Figure 6). We see that the sequential strategy of ETT followed by RNS would be acceptable as long as we were willing to spend up to $39,400 to save a year of life. The additional resources required to implement a screening strategy based on RNS as the primary screen would be acceptable if we were willing or able to spend up to $61,900 to save a year of life. However, the total resource costs of screening all asymptomatic persons over the age of 40 in the U.S., and operating on those with multiple-vessel operable disease, would be between 40 and 100 billion dollars, or between 15 and 40 percent of the total health care budget! If the results of this analysis are accepted as valid, how tenable is the position that it is desirable, or even possible, to spend an unlimited amount to save a year of life?

4.   Mild Hypertension
     (Weinstein and Stason, 1976)

The final example moves us closer to the realm of pre-

Table 1: **Alternative screening strategies in asymptomatic patients (Fineberg and Stason, in press)**

1. ANG, IF MVD ➝ SURG
2. RNS, IF ⊕ ➝ ANG, IF MVD ➝ SURG
3. ETT, IF ⊕ ➝ ANG, IF MVD ➝ SURG
4. RNS, IF ⊕ ➝ ETT, IF ⊕ ➝ ANG, IF MVD ➝ SURG
5. ETT, IF ⊕ ➝ RNS, IF ⊕ ➝ ANG, IF MVD ➝ SURG
6. DO NOTHING - OBSERVE

ANG = CORONARY ANGIOGRAPHY
MVD = MULTIPLE-VESSEL CORONARY DISEASE
SURG = CORONARY ARTERY BYPASS SURGERY
ETT = EXERCISE TOLERANCE TEST
RNS = RADIONUCLIDE SCAN

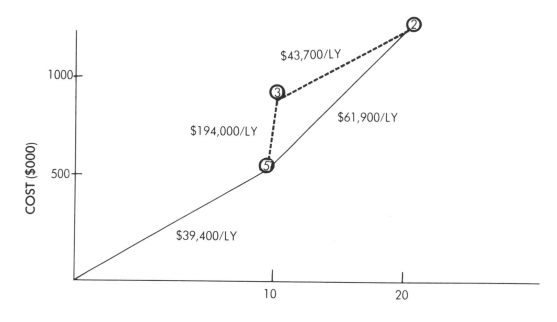

LIFE YEARS GAINED
(PRESENT VALUE)

Figure 6. Incremental costs and benefits of strategies for screening 1000 asymptomatic patients for coronary artery disease.

Strategy 2: Radionuclide scanning
Strategy 3: Exercise tolerance testing
Strategy 5: Exercise tolerance testing, followed by radionuclide scanning if positive

vention.   How cost-effective is it to avoid the occurrence of cardiovascular disease in the first place?   Among the most strongly advocated preventive measures, and one that has been validated in randomized trials, is detection and treatment of hypertension.   Particular interest has been applied to mild hypertension--diastolic blood pressures in the range of 90 to 105 mmHg--since perhaps 20 to 25 percent of the population fall into this range.

Methods.   Health care costs in the analysis included the lifetime costs of antihypertensive treatment, plus the costs of treating side effects, less any savings in the treatment of strokes or myocardial infarctions.

Effects on life expectancy were calculated based on data from the Framingham Heart Study, and assuming that a fraction of the excess risk could be eliminated by treatment.

Adjustments for the quality of life reflected the prevention of nonfatal strokes and myocardial infarctions, and adverse drug side effects.

The failure of patients to adhere to treatment can further compromise the cost-effectiveness of treatment.   In some calculations, incomplete adherence was incorporated by assuming an adherence rate of 50 percent, as experienced in the United States.

Results.   For moderate to severe hypertension, that is, diastolic pressures above 105 mmHg, with full adherence to therapy, the net cost per quality-adjusted year of life, in 1976 dollars, is only $4,850 (Figure 7).   This figure increases, however, to $10,500 when problems with adherence are introduced.   For mild hypertension between 95 and 104 mmHg, the ratio is $20,400 per quality-adjusted life year with expected adherence. For borderline hypertension in the range around 90 mmHg, the ratio is $39,600.   In 1981 dollars, the expected costs per quality-adjusted year of life saved are estimated to be $16,900 for diastolic pressures above 105 mmHg, $32,800 for mild hypertension, and $63,700 for borderline hypertension.

Screening introduces additional costs and additional problems of patient referral and follow-up (Table 2).   Based on the age-specific blood pressure distribution in the U.S., the cost per year of life gained by community-wide screening is estimated to range, in 1981 dollars, from $13,200 if full

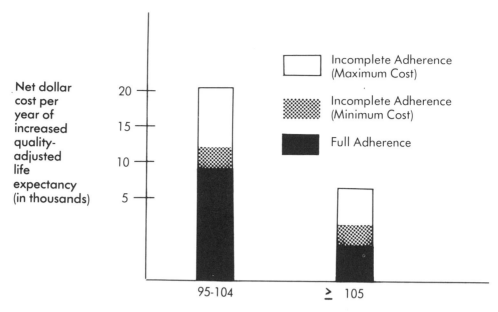

Figure 7. Cost-effectiveness of treating mild and moderate to severe hypertension, according to degree of adherence

(Source: Stason and Weinstein, 1977)

Table 2: **Cost-effectiveness of community screening for hypertension (Weinstein and Stason, 1976)**

Program	Cost per quality-adjusted year of life gained, in 1981 dollars*
SCREEN, TREAT IF DBP 95 mm Hg	
FULL ADHERENCE	13,200
EXPECTED ADHERENCE	28,700
WITH PROADHERENCE INTERVENTION	20,900
SCREEN, TREAT TO OPTIMIZE COST-EFFECTIVENESS	
FULL ADHERENCE	8,400
EXPECTED ADHERENCE	19,300
WITH PROADHERENCE INTERVENTION	12,600

*ASSUMES AN AVERAGE ANNUAL INCREASE OF 10 PERCENT IN PRICE LEVELS BETWEEN 1976 and 1981.

adherence to therapy were assumed, to $28,700 with expected adherence. This figure assumes that the threshold for treatment is 95 mmHg, for all ages and both sexes. If instead the treatment criteria by age and sex are varied to optimize cost-effectiveness of screening, the cost-effectiveness ratio falls to $19,300.

The cost-effectiveness approach may also be used to evaluate interventions intended to improve adherence. The cost effectiveness of screening for hypertension, with such an intervention in place, is estimated to be between $12,600 and $20,900, depending on the criterion for treatment.

5.   Comparison of Cost-Effectiveness Results

The results of these analyses for surgical treatment, diagnosis, screening, and prevention of coronary artery disease are summarized in Figure 8. Coronary artery bypass surgery for left-main or triple-vessel disease is the most cost-effective intervention having the lowest net cost per quality-adjusted year of life expectancy gained. Surgery for double-vessel disease is about as cost-effective as treatment of moderate to severe hypertension, and surgery for single-vessel disease is of comparable cost-effectiveness to screening for coronary disease using exercise tolerance testing confirmed by a radionuclide scan, screening for hypertension in the community, or treating mild hypertension. Treatment of borderline hypertension and screening for coronary disease by radionuclide scanning or angiography are not very cost effective.

Promises and Limitations of Cost-Effectiveness Analysis

Some examples of recent cost-effectiveness studies relating to interventions for coronary artery disease have been presented. Lest the impression is left that the only subject matter for such studies is heart disease and that the only authors are at Harvard, I would like to cite some data on the diffusion of cost-effectiveness and cost-benefit analysis in the published literature. According to a review by the Office of Technology Assessment (OTA), 421 cost effectiveness studies were published between 1966 and 1978, increasing from five in 1966 to 71 in 1978 (OTA, 1980). Informal scanning of recent journals suggests that this trend is continuing.

More than half of the studies reviewed by the OTA were published in medical journals. This is significant, because

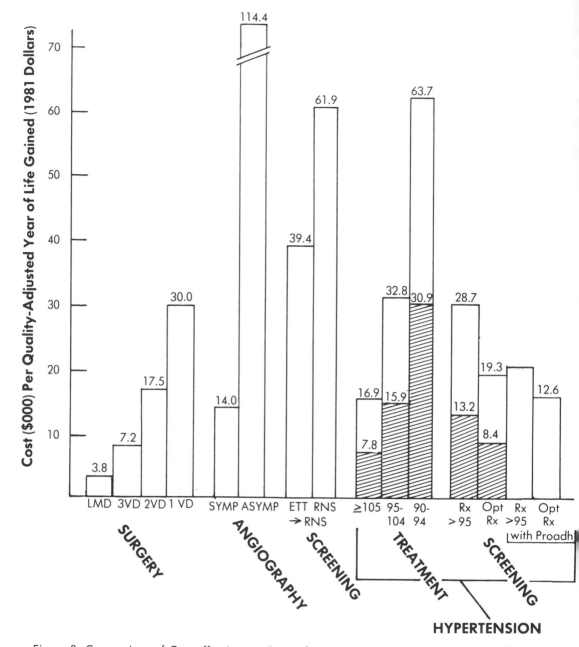

Figure 8. Comparison of Cost-effectiveness Ratios for Interventions in Coronary Artery Disease

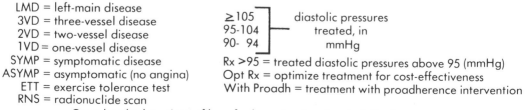

LMD = left-main disease
3VD = three-vessel disease
2VD = two-vessel disease
1VD = one-vessel disease
SYMP = symptomatic disease
ASYMP = asymptomatic (no angina)
ETT = exercise tolerance test
RNS = radionuclide scan

≥105 ⎤ diastolic pressures
95-104 ⎬ treated, in
90- 94 ⎦ mmHg
Rx >95 = treated diastolic pressures above 95 (mmHg)
Opt Rx = optimize treatment for cost-effectiveness
With Proadh = treatment with proadherence intervention

Cross-hatched portions of bars for hypertension denote full adherence it reflects greater acceptance by the medical profession of the need to take cost into account in medical decision making, and because it suggests a particular model of rationing limited resources. That model is one that retains the physician, or health care provider, as the gatekeeper of the resources , but in an environment of economic constraints or incentives; that is, an environment in which the physician is compelled to act in a cost-effective manner. In the U.S., such an environment does not yet exist, except in certain settings such as health maintenance organizations. But even in societies where resource caps are explicit, cost-effectiveness analysis has not yet had the impact that might have been expected of it, given the increasing exposure it has received. Why is that, and, more generally, what are the limitations of cost-effectiveness analysis?

First, lack of good data on efficacy means that uncertainty about costs and benefits is unavoidable. Sensitivity analysis can help to clarify the implications of uncertainty, but cannot eliminate it. Even clinical trials cannot be expected to provide all the needed information: because of their cost, and administrative complexity, they are best suited to testing qualitative hypotheses, not providing quantitative information. Clearly, new and innovative sources of data, and methods for achieving uniformity, consolidation, and availability of existing data are needed. These new directions may involve providers of care more directly in the data collection process, perhaps by using the reimbursement mechanism to provide incentives for uniform data reporting.

Second, as the examples presented show, values play an important role in the measurement of health benefits. Knowledge of attitudes toward the quality of life and its tradeoffs against longevity is as essential an ingredient of cost-effective resource allocation at the societal level as of individual patient care. And yet, our understanding of patients' preferences about health outcomes is limited indeed. The theoretical framework--based on quality-adjusted life years--is internally sound, and, I think, compelling, but the numbers that go into it are inevitably subjective. We need to validate ways to measure the quality of life, and attitudes toward it, and toward risk, so that cost-effectiveness studies can reflect our best understanding of what it is that people would want the health sector to maximize. Another implication is that mechanisms for resource allocation must somehow be designed so as to permit the expression of personal values and variation in the choice of medical technologies.

Third, there are a number of technical problems in cost-effectiveness methodology that are currently the subject of research. How should true costs be measured? How do we evaluate cost-effectiveness of a technology that has many different uses and effects? What is the appropriate way to discount future health outcomes?

A fourth class of limitations of the cost-effectiveness approach, which act as barriers to its implementation, includes those social values and concerns that are explicitly excluded from analysis. Among these are horizontal and in-tergenerational equity: to what extent should the health sector be responsible for assuring an equitable allocation of resources, among the members of society, present and future? Also in this class are political factors, such as the perceived value of a highly visible public screening program even if it is not as cost-effective as a less visible program working through individual providers. Legal factors, such as concern over liability in immunization programs, also mitigate the usefulness of analysis.

Despite these limitations, cost-effectiveness analysis, while it ought never to be used as the sole basis for a physician's decision or a regulatory action, has an impor-tant role to play in clarifying the issues surrounding medical technologies, both new and existing. By forcing explicit assumptions but permitting sensitivity analyses to explore the implications of those assumptions where the data are least secure, such analyses can have a desirable impact on the processes, if not the outcome, of health care policy making, resource allocation, and medical decision making.

Supported in part by a grant by the Robert Wood Johnson Foundation to the Center for the Analysis of Health Prac-tices.

References

Altman SH, Blendon R (eds.). 1979. Medical Technology: The Culprit Behind Health Care Costs? Washington. D.C.: Government Printing Office.

Banta HD, Behney CJ, Willems JS. 1981. Toward rational technology in medicine. New York, NY: Springer Publishing Co.

Banta HD, Thacker SB. 1979. Assessing the costs and benefits of electronic fetal monitoring. Obstet Gynecol Survey 34:627-642.

Feldstein M, Taylor, A. 1977. The rapid rise of hospital costs. Washington, D.C.: President's Council on Wage and Price Stability.

Fineberg HV. 1979. Clinical chemistries: the high cost of low-cost diagnostic tests. In (Altman SH, Blendon, R eds.) Medical Technology: The Culprit Behind Health Care Costs. Washington, D.C.: Government Printing Office.

Fineberg HV, Stason WB. In press. Cost-effectiveness of alternative diagnostic strategies for coronary artery disease. Circulation.

Freeland M, Calat G, Schendler CE. 1980. Projections of national health expenditures, 1980, 1985, and 1990. Health Care Financing Review 1:1-27.

Kaplan RM, Bush JW, Berry CC. 1976. Health status: types of validity and the index of well-being. Health Services Research 11:478-507.

Office of Technology Assessment. U.S. Congress. 1978a. Assessing the efficacy and safety of medical technologies. Washington, D.C.: Government Printing Office.

Office of Technology Assessment. U.S. Congress. 1978b. Policy implications of the computed tomography (CT) scanner. Washington, D.C.: Government Printing Office.

Office of Technology Assessment. U.S. Congress. 1980. The implications of cost-effectiveness alanysis of medical technology. Washington, D.C.: Government Printing Office.

Scitovsky A, McCall N. 1976. Changes in the costs of treatment of selected illnesses, 1951-1964-1971. DHEW Publication No. (HRA) 77-361. Washington. D.C.: National Center for Health Services Research.

Stason WB, Weinstein MC. 1977. Allocation of resources to manage hypertension. N Engl J Med 296:732-739.

Torrance GW. 1976. Social preferences for health states: an empirical evaluation of three measurement techniques. Socio-Economic Planning Sciences 10:129-136.

United States Department of Health and Human Services. 1980. Health United States 1980. Hyattsville, MD: Government Printing Office.

Weinstein MC. 1981. Economic assessments of medical practices and technologies. Medical Decision Making 1:309-330.

Weinstein MC, Pearlman LA. 1981. Cost-effectiveness of automated multichannel chemistry analyzers. Case study number 4. In (Office of Technology Assessment) Cost-Effectiveness Analysis of Medical Technology. Washington, D.C.: Government Printing Office.

Weinstein MC, Stason WB. 1976. Hypertension: a policy perspective. Cambridge, MA: Harvard University Press.

Weinstein MC, Stason WB. 1977. Foundations of cost-effectiveness analysis for health and medical practices. N Engl J Med 296:716-721.

Weinstein MC, Stason WB. In press. Cost-effectiveness of coronary artery bypass surgery. Circulation.

COMPETITION AND HEALTH CARE TECHNOLOGY: CAN WE DECENTRALIZE DECISION MAKING?
Clark C. Havighurst, J.D.

Health policy discussions can miss the mark for many reasons, but a particular failing in most discussions of the issues presented by new and existing health care technology has been the prevalence of the assumption that our methods for paying for health services will remain as dysfunctional in the future as they have been in the past. Often this assumption has led to automatic acceptance of the idea that technology questions must be addressed on some collective or centralized basis--either through government regulation or through formal or informal processes sponsored by the medical care industry itself. Perhaps the main point of this paper is that the emergence of the so-called competition strategy in the national health policy debate makes it inappropriate to assume that the range of policy options is limited to a choice among various mechanisms of centralized decision making. Indeed, the overriding objective of introducing competition into the financing and delivery of health services would be to bring consumers' cost-consciousness to bear on providers in new ways, thus permitting reliance on diverse and unspecified institutions of private decision making to allocate resources to and within the health care sector.

Historical Background of the Competition Strategy

Some historical and political background will show where the idea of competition came from and why it currently enjoys some policymakers' support. As recently as 1978, competition was almost exclusively an academic idea, and the conventional wisdom was that government, one way or another, would have to control health care costs through regulation. Competition was simply a code word for encouraging the development of health maintenance organizations (HMOs) as part of a pluralistic but still largely noncompetitive system. The fee-for-service sector itself was viewed as immune to internal price competition and able to weather a great deal of HMO competition without having to change its spend-thrift ways. This imperviousness to competition was deemed to result from providers' presumed ability to create their own demand. The Carter administration, viewing the challenge as one of designing regulation to curb these cost-escalating tendencies, came up with its hospital cost containment bill in 1977. Even though it was a logical extension of the trend toward regulation, that bill to limit arbitrarily the growth of hospital revenues never made it through the Congress.

Assumptions about the inevitability of regulation began seriously to break down in 1979 when the 96th Congress convened. With its defeat of the Carter cap proposal in late 1979, Congress effectively seized the policy initiative from HEW (now HHS), which had nothing left to offer once the centerpiece of its program was lost. Several individual members of Congress moved into the resulting policy vacuum, including most of the leaders of the congressional fight against hospital cost containment. Even though the defeat of that legislation was widely credited to effective industry lobbying, in fact it owed a great deal to the willingness of Congress first to think through the full implications of further pursuit of regulation and then to recognize a market-oriented alternative to the kind of heavy-handed regulation that the Carter proposal contemplated. Thus, the leaders in the fight against the Carter bill, particularly Congressmen Gephardt, Stockman, and Jones and Senators Schweiker and Durenberger, took seriously their responsibility for coming up with an alternative solution to the cost problem and subsequently sponsored bills to reform the health care marketplace. In addition to these substantial contributions to the appearance of the market strategy, the 96th Congress also enacted the health planning amendments of 1979, which included the first legislative endorsement of competition as a potentially desirable force in the health care field.

Political Trends Favoring the Competition Strategy

The emergence of the competition strategy was probably inevitable, even though few people foresaw the force with which it would enter the policy debate. The movement toward deregulation in other industries should have indicated that it was just a matter of time before Congress's right hand would realize what its left hand had been doing in the health care industry. Moreover, it should have been obvious that the new forms of regulation needed to achieve effective cost control in the health sector would be intolerably arbitrary and insensitive, systematically evading (or shifting to providers) the difficult choices which are necessarily involved in rationing health care but which government cannot afford to face on a case-by-case basis. The mild forms of regulation that Congress had been willing to tolerate were producing virtually no measurable results, and the new prescriptions were distinctly unpalatable.

As regulation was disappointing expectations and losing favor, the arguments for competition were gaining force as a result of able advocacy, particularly the appearance of Alain Enthoven's Consumer-Choice Health Plan, which gave concreteness to what had previously been only an abstract theory. By focusing on the key principle of cost-conscious consumer choice, the Enthoven plan also helped to shift the debate away from an exclusive focus on HMOs. At the same time, continued experience with HMO-inspired competition, in Minneapolis-St. Paul and elsewhere, was helping to advance the flag of competition in the public debate. Finally, the antitrust enforcement effort and the Federal Trade Commission's emergence as competition's first liberal advocate-- and its first advocate of any kind within the federal establishment--gave competition new credibility and respectability.

Subtle changes in public attitudes toward health and health care also contributed to the emergence of the competition strategy. The increasing emphasis in recent years on personal responsibility for one's own health has coincided with the reduced frequency of references to the "right to health care." One implication of this shift in attitudes is greater acceptance of the idea that people can be expected to bear some of the cost of their own health care and can be allowed to make cost-conscious choices. Evidence that health services vary widely in their efficacy and cost effectiveness and that personal health care is not always the most important contributor to improved health status has likewise increased tolerance for diversity and consumer choice.

Yet another factor that brought competition back into the policy debate was the disappearance of the more extreme models of national health insurance. Because early proposals contemplated that government would serve as the great third-party payer, health policy concentrated on perfecting government's tools for policing the system and neglected private financing mechanisms and consumer choice, which were seen as vestiges of the past shortly to be displaced. Thus, the policy agenda changed dramatically when Senator Kennedy and the labor movement agreed in the mid-1970s to accept a role for private health insurers, as well as HMOs, in the projected national health insurance system. Suddenly it became necessary to consider how to get good performance from the private sector, and competition was undeniably a viable contender for a substantial role in that effort. Indeed, once the issue was posed in this way, competition began to look quite promising in comparison to regulation.

The advent of the Reagan administration appears, of course, to have increased the chances that pro-competition legislation will ultimately be enacted. Obviously, the proponents of market-reform bills have moved into prominent positions, and there have been several expressions of a commitment to pursue the strategy actively. It is worth noting, however, that the competition strategy was already established in Washington and had some real momentum behind it, before the Reagan administration came to town. Moreover, it is not exclusively or even predominantly a Republican initiative. Indeed, although HEW-HHS in the Carter years would not hear of these ideas, others in the Carter administration took a substantial interest in them. In particular (though he was not alone), Alfred Kahn--the patron saint of deregulators--was vigorously promoting the competition strategy when the Carter administration left office. In addition, there are many other signs, such as the Gephardt-Stockman bill, that the market strategy could turn out to be a bipartisan effort. Indeed, as they did with deregulation, the Democrats might ultimately make this initiative their own, and, in some respects, they might prove more capable of carrying it out in a responsible way--particularly by paying adequate attention to some of the side effects on poor people that the administration may be inclined to neglect. Just as only a Republican administration could open the door to China, perhaps only the Democrats will eventually be able to carry out a fully developed market-oriented policy in health care.

Even though the political climate now seems hospitable to a market-oriented national health policy, government may not be able to follow all the way through in implementing a pro-competitive strategy. Antagonism toward regulation is

not the same thing as favoring aggressive efforts to rehabilitate the market as a force for changing the status quo.
Indeed, a philosophical commitment to reducing government's
role could easily undercut such necessary measures as antitrust enforcement and the provision of new public funds to
replace desirable internal subsidies eroded by competition.
Similarly, a philosophical disposition to return responsibilities to the states invites the continuation of regulatory patterns and state-supported professional controls that
have long diminished competition's force. Finally, government has great difficulty in pursuing any goal singlemindedly
through the thickets of special interests. Recent history
suggests that the federal government may be chronically un-
able to settle on a coherent and internally consistent
national health policy and to implement it on all fronts.
I am not yet persuaded that the nation has, or can ever get,
the leadership necessary to act forthrightly and consistently
on this extremely important subject.

Where the Competition Strategy Stands Today

In the current Congress, there are several bills that embody
elements of a competition strategy. The Gephardt-Stockman
bill (H.R. 850) is the most ambitious one, resembling in
many respects the comprehensive plan developed by Professor
Enthoven. Under it, the federal government would offer a
menu of qualified health plans from which all citizens would
ultimately be free to choose. Premiums up to a fixed amount
would be subsidized through the tax system or otherwise,
but incentives to economize would also exist. This bill
amounts to a national health insurance plan and would funda-
mentally transform the Medicare and Medicaid programs into
voucher-type schemes. Among the other pro-competition
bills, Senator Durenberger's (S. 433) contemplates capping
the tax-free treatment of employer contributions to private
health plans and would prevent large employers from offering
only a single health plan, requiring instead the offering of
"multiple choice" (at least three plans) and an equal dollar
contribution to whichever plan the employee chooses, so that
employees will see opportunities to economize. Senator
Hatch's bill (S. 139) is essentially the one introduced by
Secretary Schweiker in the last Congress. It also would require large employers to offer multiple choice, including a
plan with extensive cost sharing, and would allow employees
choosing a low-cost plan to receive the premium saving as
non-taxable income. Several other proposals have focused
on the Medicare program and the possibility of allowing bene-
ficiaries to enroll at government expense in an HMO or per-

haps in some other kind of private health plan.

None of the pending pro-competition bills, with the possible exception of the Medicare-HMO option, is receiving what may be regarded as really serious legislative attention at this time.   This lack of current activity results largely from the Reagan administration's failure to introduce its promised contender into the field.   Although the HHS staff has labored hard, many decisions remain to be made.   The most likely prospect is for the administration to offer a bill, or perhaps two or more bills, early in 1982.   The package is likely to limit the tax subsidy for employer-paid premiums (perhaps by limiting the employer's deduction rather than by taxing the employee) and to permit tax-free rebates (up to some maximum amount) for additional economizing under the tax cap.   The administration is not likely to propose mandatory multiple choice which has been increasingly recognized as a new and potentially burdensome form of regulation that would probably not be necessary if a meaningful tax change were made.   The administration will also probably indicate a strong desire to introduce the principle of consumer choice into the Medicare program, but technical and cost problems may prevent it from going as far in this direction as it would like.

There would seem to be only limited prospects for action on any of these proposals in the present Congress, but the possibility should not be ruled out.   In the midst of the current concern about budget deficits, the idea of imposing a limitation on the tax subsidy for private insurance may look particularly attractive to Congress as a revenue-raising measure that also advances an important policy objective.   While controversial, the tax change may still be the easiest of the proposals to sell in Congress.

Decision Making on Technology Issues Under Competition

The market strategy contemplates making certain changes in consumers' incentives and widening their opportunities for choice in the market for health care financing plans and health care services.   The theory is that new consumer cost-consciousness will increase competitive pressures for innovation in private financing mechanisms.   The resulting changes in financing arrangements are expected to facilitate the transmission of consumers' cost concerns, in one way or another, to providers, forcing them into price- and cost-reducing competition and thus changing behavior in desirable ways throughout the system.   I share the view that, if we

can get incentives and competitive conditions right, technology problems could be expected largely to take care of
themselves.   Although there would still be a need for public
subsidies to support technology assessment and the development and dissemination of new knowledge, there is no substantial reason not to entrust the choices that are to be
made in light of that knowledge to private decision makers.
Thus, I would argue that the issues presented by the introduction and use of technology should not be distinguished
too sharply from other issues confronting the health care
industry.   In particular, the problem of health care costs
should be understood as not just a concern that costs are
somehow "too high" but as a concern about the inefficiency
of our mechanisms for allocating health resources, technology
included.

In order to understand the potential, as well as the
limitations, of the market-oriented approach to technology
issues, it is necessary to consider some of the mechanisms
by which the competitive market could translate consumers'
wishes into roughly appropriate provider behavior in employing technology. The mechanism that most obviously and readily lends itself to this purpose is the HMO, particularly
the prepaid group practice.   In an HMO, providers of care,
constrained by the necessity to set a competitive premium,
must make choices about the capital investments to make, the
nature, the quality, and quantity of manpower and equipment
to employ, and the utilization to be made of existing resources.   Physicians in such an organized system would be
inclined to employ those technologies in which they have the
most confidence and to await demonstrations of the efficacy
of new technologies.   Implicit systems of rationing would be
employed so that only those patients likely to benefit substantially from the use of existing technology would be given
access to it.   On the other hand, the necessity to maintain
consumer loyalty and the plan's reputation for providing
good-quality care would prevent such plans from withholding
valuable treatments.   Despite consumers' imperfect ability
to evaluate the trade-offs between premiums and the plan's
policies toward technology and other factors, the general
tendency under free competition would be toward optimal use
of technology and optimal levels of health care spending.
Because plans could hardly expect to succeed for long if they
consistently disappointed consumer expectations with respect
to either cost or quality, a market consisting of a variety
of competing closed-panel HMOs would not require much su-
pervision with respect to choices regarding technology.

Questions may be asked, however, concerning that portion of the market which is not organized into competing organized delivery systems, such as HMOs. One important element in the competition strategy is, of course, the expectation that competitive forces will drive more and more consumers and providers into organized systems. Not all of these systems need be HMOs, however, and one can anticipate a wide variety of plans, many of them modeled after traditional insurance plans, having the capacity to guide providers toward more appropriate use of resources. Where the chosen plan does not restrict the consumer's choice of provider, cost-containment efforts would have to take the form of explicit coverage limitations forcing consumers to spend their own money on questionable procedures or on increments of care or quality having only marginal value. Although one might doubt the marketability of plans that attempt minutely to define the insured's right to be treated using various technologies, that option is at least available. For example, a plan might limit coverage of coronary bypass surgery, either excluding it as a benefit altogether (on the ground that it has not been shown to have lifesaving value) or requiring heavy cost sharing. A plan also might limit its obligation to pay for CT scans in the absence of specific indications, which the physician would have to certify; if physician certifications were thought unreliable for such screening purposes, the plan might restrict the providers who were eligible to prescribe, or provide, covered scans.

There are no doubt numerous other ways in which health plans might explicitly or implicitly ration either services or the availability of funds. My purpose is not to appraise the desirability or marketability or administrative feasibility of these various strategies but only to point out that the marketplace, under reinstated incentives, would have reason to develop and enforce new controls on spending. If traditional insurance plans could not adapt themselves, they would be replaced by HMOs or other plans that did possess a cost-containment capability. It is, of course, not clear how many consumers would be willing to pay the high premiums of plans that offered virtually unlimited and costless access to high-cost technology.

I strongly believe that the private sector, employing imperfect techniques of the kinds previously sketched, offers the best mechanisms we can hope to find for facing the sometimes tragic choices that medical care necessarily presents to people. Our long experience with regulation has shown, I think, that government inherently lacks the power to deal successfully with sensitive trade-offs.   Competition and consumer choice, on the other hand, seem to me to have powerful inherent advantages in dealing with such issues. The market can, and does, find ways of presenting choices to consumers in more or less manageable forms, either explicitly or implicitly.   Consumers are thus allowed to register their preferences and to give some effect to their reluctance to underwrite expensive practices that are unproved or undesirable or insufficiently beneficial from their point of view.   Although the market has inherent limitations of its own--due primarily to consumers' ignorance and inability to make fine risk-benefit calculations--there is clearly a wide range within which choice can safely be allowed to operate. The market strategy, as I and others have outlined it, provides plenty of opportunities for consumers to pool their resources and knowledge and to employ knowledgeable and trustworthy agents to help them choose.   Technology questions would be among those that providers would have to address with the knowledge that their choices would have to be acceptable to consumers who had the option of taking their business elsewhere.

Because the ultimate decisions in a competitive system would be made by cost-conscious consumers and not by non-accountable professionals, it should come as no surprise if what passes for the quality of care, as judged by professional standards, should decline somewhat in a competitive world.   Alain Enthoven argues forcefully that competition will improve quality--recall, for example, his Shattuck Lecture at Harvard entitled "Cutting Costs Without Cutting the Quality of Care"--and I am quite convinced by his argument that there would indeed be a net quality gain.   But I would not concede, as he seems to do, that that is the issue.   Because I think that people are entitled to economize on "quality" in health care and to spend their money on other things, I would be fully prepared to accept a decline in quality.   Indeed, I would specifically expect to find that, by some measures at least, quality is too high in many parts of the system which the medical establishment has designed and that the net gains anticipated by Enthoven are the result of substantial improvements in professionally neglected areas that outweigh distinct losses in others.   In any event, the issue is not whether the quality of care might decline somewhat, or somewhere, in a competitive system but whether people in general will be better off.   As a general rule, what people save by economizing will be worth more to them than any services or increments of quality that they give up. I know of no better way of facing the difficult choices that technology presents to us than to let people choose for themselves.

Will Society Tolerate Economizing Choices?

You will recall that I argued at the outset that policy discussions of technology questions can miss the mark by assuming the incapacity of private decision-making mechanisms. One can also go wrong by assuming too readily that private institutions are free and uninhibited in addressing hard choices of the sort with which health care technology confronts us. The purpose of these final comments is to suggest that it will not be easy to shift decision-making responsibility on technology questions to the competitive private sector and that specific attention must therefore be given to removing unnecessary restrictions on private discretion. In fact, society imposes a number of constraints, both formal and informal, on the freedom of private decision makers to make choices on the delicate matters involved in deploying and using costly health care technology. Through its legal and regulatory institutions, society has sometimes prescribed the terms of dealing on such issues. Even where it has not specifically prescribed terms in advance, it has sometimes shown itself unwilling to accept and enforce bargains that are freely struck by the private parties but later regretted by one of them. While this is not the place to provide a definitive analysis, I want at least to suggest some areas where reforms not usually contemplated by pro-competition strategists may be needed before we can be certain that private choices can effectively displace collective, professional, or other centralized controls.

The problem, as I see it, exists on two levels. One set of problems lies within the medical care sector itself, where there is little acceptance of the notion of diversity or of the idea that departures from common norms may sometimes, for cost reasons, be desirable rather than undesirable. The other set of problems lies within our legal institutions, which no longer venerate freedom of contract and now often impose on contracting parties, particularly those perceived as economically powerful, duties inconsistent with their contractually specified obligations. In the case of both sets of obstacles to privately sponsored innovation, we are looking at expressions of fundamental societal mores that, while they may provide no absolute barriers to widening the scope of private decision making, certainly inhibit the effective redesign of private insurance and the development of other independent solutions to the difficult trade-offs with which medical care abounds. There are, in fact, numerous reasons to believe that many efficiency-dictated reductions in the cost and quality of inputs employed in medical and hospital care, in utilization levels, and in the availability of insurance coverage for desirable but non-essential services are currently inhibited by much more than just the system's weak cost-consciousness. Thus, policy measures strengthening the latter may fail to trigger the former. At least, the expectation that private choices will be allowed to freely guide the system must be tempered with recognition that there are serious countervailing factors.

Obviously, a full review of these large questions would require a treatise probing not only the legal and regulatory institutions of our society but also the mores that underlie them. For present purposes, I can only mention a few of the specific obstacles to the kinds of changes that I would regard as ultimately necessary to ensure that the private market will approach optimal resource allocation and appropriately discipline the development and use of health care technology.

Within the medical care sector, one source of the problem lies in the common conception that medical care is a science exact enough to be reducible to rules and amenable to central control. A badly needed attitudinal reform in the health care industry is the rejection of the notion that there is a single right way, or a narrow range of acceptable ways, to diagnose and treat human disease that must somehow be established and enforced on a collective basis, either by the medical profession or by the government. Instead of perpetuating this misconception, we need to establish the legitimacy of pluralistic approaches within a wide range, using public controls and professional self-regulation only to address problems bordering on misrepresentation and exploitation.

The concept of a unitary standard of care appears at various points in the medical care system. One significant example is the concept of "medical necessity" that is embodied in the Professional Standards Review Organization (PSRO) program and in professional peer review mechanisms of all kinds. The assumption underlying the PSRO program seems to be that there is some objective professional consensus, some scientific concept of right and wrong, that should determine the appropriateness of federal payments for medical and hospital services. Private health insurers, too, have very often accepted the medical profession's concept that it knows best what should be paid for, and, of late, we are hearing the involvement of PSROs in claims review for private health plans hailed as a positive development. In addition to thinking that a PSRO would run serious antitrust risks in extending its services outside its statutory sphere, I regret the loss of opportunities for private health plans to assume responsibility for setting their own limits on what they will pay for. This suggestion that insurers, rather than the medical profession, should be the ultimate arbiter of what should be paid for will strike most of this audience as radical, but that reaction simply demonstrates just how far we are from fully accepting the notion of consumer choice. Until the legitimacy of decentralized decision making on coverage questions is fully established, the private market will be restrained in dealing with technology questions. It is perhaps worth noting that we do already accept implicit limitations on coverage to the extent that we tolerate HMOs' conservative policy toward hospitalization and otherwise let HMOs define their own standards.

Another illustration of our commitment to a unitary standard of medical care is malpractice law, which embodies a community standard of care and enforces that standard with considerable rigor. Thus, an HMO seeking to economize in a specific and responsible way must be concerned that, if it departs from customary practice, it will be held liable for any bad outcome that might occur. Because the standards of customary practice have been developed in a market largely unconstrained by cost considerations, the malpractice system is enforcing a demonstrably inefficient and inappropriate standard. Thus, it stands as a significant deterrent to many of the kinds of privately initiated economizing that market strategists are hoping to encourage.

In order to illustrate some of the issues discussed let me describe a conversation I once participated in with an HMO administrator. The administrator reported that his plan felt compelled to provide fetal monitoring for all pregnant women because that was the standard of care prevailing in the community. (Alain Enthoven, who was also there, observed at this point that this practice was not good medicine because fetal monitoring has been shown to be of no benefit and some risk in a majority of cases. I preferred not to take this easy way out, however, and pressed on with the idea that the service should be dispensed with wherever it is not worth its cost.) The discussion then focused on how the HMO could alter its practice without paying a malpractice claim whenever a jury thought a bad outcome might have been prevented. After we considered some malpractice defenses that might work, the question arose whether the HMO's subscriber contract could be written to exclude the service; we doubted whether that fine print would be enough to deter a court from imposing liability. We then considered whether the consumer advisory panel which the plan maintained might be asked to approve the omission of the service in appropriate cases, an action which might add legitimacy to a specific provision in the contract. Another thought was that the HMO might by contract exclude the service as a covered benefit but offer it, with full disclosure, to those who might wish to pay the cost. This, of course, would violate the HMO's ideological commitment to providing a single style of prepaid care, yet it seemed a good way of introducing appropriate diversity and expanding patients' opportunities for choice.

This example presents several lessons. The misdirected influence of the malpractice system is clear, and the limitations of private decision makers in helping consumers to escape the law's inappropriate standards are also demonstrated. To my mind, the case also illustrates the desirability of limiting coverage without denying consumers the right to spend their own money on services that they might choose with their physician's advice.

The case also suggests the difficulty that the courts would have in giving full effect to provisions in an HMO's subscriber contract that might turn out to impose a hardship on an individual consumer. California courts have been willing to enforce arbitration clauses in HMOs' collectively bargained subscriber contracts, thus indicating that individuals will sometimes be allowed to give up certain "rights" pursuant to contractual understandings. It seems more doubtful, however, that they would be permitted to waive altogether their right to sue physicians for malpractice. Such waivers were proposed a few years ago by Professor Richard Epstein of the University of Chicago Law School, who argued that the reduction in fees that patients would enjoy would be more than adequate compensation for the additional risks that they would bear. I have myself considered the possibility that a no-fault compensation scheme might be offered by an HMO or other organized health plan as an exclusive remedy for certain predefined injuries that its patients might suffer. Whether such a scheme would be enforced by the courts is an open question, though if it were developed freely and with consumer input and had some additional legitimacy attached by virtue of an insurance commissioner's approval, it might well stand the judicial test. Comparable questions of enforceability would also arise if insurers sought to limit their payment responsibilities for care in some of the many gray areas. Unless reasonable coverage limitations are enforced, private decision making cannot serve as our guide to the goal of an efficient allocation of resources.

I have tried to show that there are in our society some unrecognized obstacles to letting private parties strike bargains that impose any risk on the allegedly uninformed consumer. Even when that consumer has benefitted by reason of a lower price and his decision was well within the bounds of rationality, regulators and judges may rush to his rescue when the risk that he assumed materializes. Because of the obstacles I have identified to the operation of a truly free market in medical care, there may be some reason to doubt that the market solution to the problems of the health care industry will bring us automatically to a cost-benefit millennium. Nevertheless, the market does not have to be entirely free--and perhaps should not be entirely free--for it still to qualify as the best mechanism we have available for addressing the difficult trade-offs presented by health care technology and by its sometimes questionable capacity to provide marginal benefits to mankind that justify incurring its marginal costs.

SOME APHORISMS CONCERNING MEDICAL TECHNOLOGY ILLUSTRATED BY SPECIFIC CASE EXAMPLES
H. David Banta, M.D., M.P.H.

Almost everyone would agree that medical technology has been very beneficial during the last several decades. Infectious disease is largely controlled in this country; dietary deficiencies are seldom seen; some cancers can be effectively treated. The pattern of disease has changed markedly since 1900, when about 50 percent of deaths were related to infectious disease. Chronic diseases predominate now.

Chronic diseases, with their multi-factorial etiologies and their long incubation periods, will not be easy to control. Many of the factors that have been identified as casually-associated with these diseases are related to individual behavior: smoking, drinking alcohol, eating fats, doing no vigorous exercise. However, there still are opportunities for technological intervention. Treatment of hypertension prevents strokes, heart attacks, and premature death. Cancer screening and early treatment could prevent many cancer deaths and chronic disease. Influenza and pneumococcal vaccines could prevent much ill-health and chronic disease, especially in the elderly. Technology can help the handicapped to become more functional and in many cases self-supporting.

The problem is apparent to everyone. The rising costs of health care have made us realize that resources available for health care are limited. We are already ignoring significant opportunities for improving the health of our people. As costs continue to rise, the situation can only worsen.

Thus, this paper will look at problems associated with

medical technology. I define technology as "science applied to a definite goal." Medical technology includes drugs, devices, and procedures, as well as aggregations into systems such as intensive care units and even hospitals. Technology is neither good nor bad in itself. If the goal is well-defined, and people agree that it is worthwhile, then there apparently is no serious problem. However, technology is also diverse, and it is difficult to generalize. Technology and its use have broad-ranging consequences. Hopefully, some cases will illustrate a set of aphorisms and give an indication of what our problems really are.

Aphorism One

<u>While medical technology is unquestionably a major contribution to rising health care costs, it is not easy to characterize which technology is the problem.</u>

According to economic analyses, technology has accounted for 33-75 percent of the rise in hospital costs. However, this figure is difficult to associate with specific technologies.

The national health care expenditure was $212 billion in 1979. The largest one portion is hospital care, making up 40 percent. An estimated 10-15 percent of that is intensive care, itself a complex of technologies.

Diagnostic imaging costs this country about $10 billion a year, with diagnostic x-ray making up about $7.6 billion of the total. Diagnostic laboratory services cost $15-20 billion a year. Diagnostic tests have been found in themselves to account for up to 40 percent of the increase in hospital costs.

In contrast, widely publicized capital intensive technologies contribute smaller percentages. CT scanners ($875 million), coronary bypass surgery ($1.5 billion) and electronic fetal monitoring ($411 million) do not make a ripple in the figures.

It seems clear that controlling visible, capital intensive technologies will not control costs. On the other hand, how can we control the 5 billion or more lab tests performed in this country in a year?

Aphorism Two

Diffusion (spread) into use of new medical technologies is often so rapid that adequate testing for efficacy and safety cannot be done in time to influence diffusion and distribution.

The computed tomography (CT) scanner is the prototype example of rapid diffusion. First introduced into the United States in 1973, with a price of about $350,000, it was rapidly accepted. (Figure 1). By May 1980, there were 1,471 scanners. During 1978, about 40 scanners a month were installed, representing a capital investment per month of about $20 million. This rapid diffusion occurred in the absence of careful evaluation. By June 1975 there were almost 100 scanners, but only 13 clinical papers had been published.

That the diffusion rate was indeed rapid may be demonstrated in a variety of ways. One is to compare the U.S. experience with that of other countries. By early 1979, the U.S. had 5.7 scanners per million persons, the largest number of scanners per capita in the world. That figure may be compared with West Germany (2.6), France (0.6), Sweden (1.7), and so forth.

Another way of gauging the rapidity of diffusion is to examine other similar technologies. Radionuclide scanning came into widespread use in the 1950s. During the period 1952 to 1969 it diffused at the rate of less than 100 per year. During the period 1969 to 1972 it diffused at the rate of almost 200 per year. The rate for both periods was lower than that for CT scanning. The different rate between the two periods also suggests that something may have changed. It is worth noting that the Medicare and Medicaid programs were enacted in 1965.

Rapid diffusion can be promoted by various factors, including situations where people are very ill and physicians have little to offer them. Figure 2, for example, shows the case of leukemia chemotherapy. Warner calls this rapid diffusion in the absence of proof of efficacy "desperation-reaction." Desperation has certainly played a part in the spread of what Thomas called "half-way" technology, technology that does not influence the disease process, but compensates for its symptoms or effects. Renal dialysis, cardiac pacemakers, and respirators are examples of such technology. These types of technology can be particularly ex-

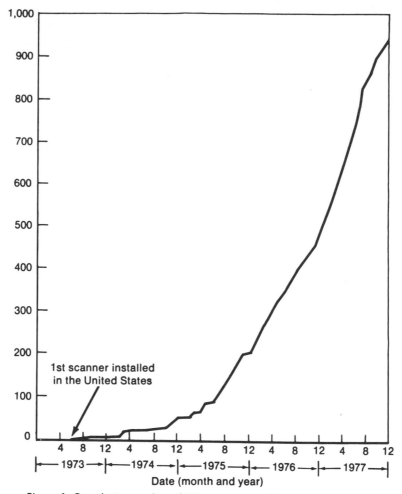

Figure 1. Cumulative number of CT scanners installed, 1973-1977

(% of Patients Treated)

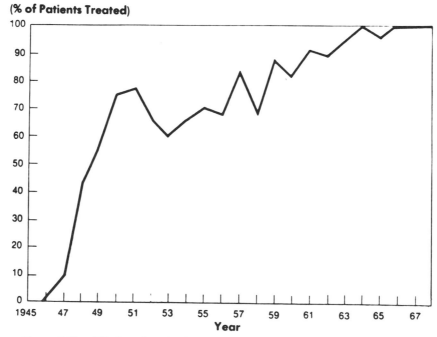

Figure 2. The diffusion of medical technologies: Chemotherapy for leukemia

pensive because once begun, they must often be used until the patient dies.

Aphorism Three

Some technologies have come into widespread use and later have been shown to lack efficacy.

Cochrane and Fineberg and Hiatt have produced lists of such technologies. The case of gastric freezing is most often quoted. Gastric freezing was developed by a prominent surgeon, Dr. Owen Wangensteen, for the treatment of peptic ulcer during the mid-1950s. Wangensteen convinced a small company, Swenko, to manufacture his device. Wangensteen presented his findings, indicating substantial clinical benefit, in 1962. His presentation created a public stir, as well as excitement in the medical profession. Thousands of patients were treated by gastric freezing; at least 1,000 devices were purchased. Subsequently, the procedure was found to be worthless as a treatment for peptic ulcer, and it also caused considerable harm. By 1966, gastric freezing had fallen out of use in the United States.

Skull x-ray for the diagnosis of skull fracture is an example still in widespread use. In 1977, an estimated 5.7 million skull x-ray examinations were carried out. An estimated 20 to 30 percent are done to evaluate head injury. Bell and Loop studied the use of skull x-rays for trauma by two hospitals. Serious injury was diagnosed by other means. Unsuspected fractures were found, but the diagnosis did not change therapy. Bell and Loop also found that 20 percent of examinations were done for "trivial injury" and that another 34 percent were done to protect against possible malpractice suits. These findings were replicated by Jergens, Morgan and McElroy.

Radical mastectomy is another technology in widespread use that does not appear to have advantages in comparison with simpler procedures. Radical mastectomy has been used as a treatment for breast cancer for about 100 years. Many such procedures are still done. However, a number of clinical trials indicate that less mutilating procedures are equally beneficial. Although there is now active controversy in the medical profession about the appropriateness of radical mastectomy, it is falling in use and will probably eventually largely disappear from surgical practice.

Some have hoped that if inefficacious technologies could be removed from practice that would solve the cost problem while improving quality of care. There do seem to be certain widespread technologies that came into practice years or even decades ago that have not been demonstrated to be efficacious. However, this does seem to be a minority of technology.

Aphorism Four

Safety is not adequately taken into account in deciding to use technology.

All technology is associated with risks, in some cases serious ones. X-rays, for example, are associated with cancer. Radical mastectomy is associated with all the risks of major surgery. Gastric freezing caused gastric ulceration and burn-like damage to gastric tissue. Coronary bypass surgery is associated with a one to two percent mortality rate, as well as other risks of surgery. Mammography screening can cause cancer, and its risk could exceed its benefit, especially in younger women.

Few physicians would choose to provide a technology that had risks if they were not convinced it also had benefits. Thus, the real problem is how to balance benefits and risks.

A good example is that of chemotherapy for lung cancer. For extensive lung cancer, chemotherapy increases survival approximately two months over that of a placebo-treated group. However, chemotherapy often affects the bone marrow, making the patient subject to infection. Nausea and loss of appetite are common. Hospitalization is usually necessary. Yet the majority of patients are treated. The complexities of this case, including the likely demise of the patient, indicate that balancing benefits and risks is not necessarily a simple matter.

Aphorism Five

Many technologies appear to be inappropriately and excessively used, based on what is known about their efficacy and safety.

Cesarean section, or Cesarean birth, was done in 4.5

percent of deliveries in the United States in 1965 and in 18 percent of deliveries in 1979. (Figure 3). This rate is probably the highest in the world. The French rate was about 8.5 percent in 1976, and the rate in The Netherlands was 2.8 percent in 1975. A recent meeting at the National Institutes of Health found the following conditions to contribute to the rising rate in this country: dystocia or cephalopelvic disproportion (30 percent), repeat Cesarean section (25-30 percent), breech delivery (10-15 percent), and fetal distress. Dystocia is criticized as a non-specific diagnosis and repeat Cesarean is not recommended in the report. It seems clear from this report that the Cesarean rate in this country is excessive. There is no information to indicate benefit from this high rate.

Another technology, electronic fetal monitoring (EFM), is associated with the inappropriate diagnosis of fetal distress, and correspondingly with inappropriate Cesarean sections. EFM is used in 60-70 percent of deliveries in the United States. There is no evidence that the true incidence of fetal distress has changed, while the diagnosis has increased. It is also worth noting the EFM has at least partially displaced auscultation, a cheaper and simpler method of monitoring the fetus. Clinical trials have failed to demonstrate benefit from routine EFM, except possibly in the low birth weight fetus, which makes up about 10 percent of deliveries.

Respiratory therapy is made up of a complex of treatments directed at maintaining, improving, or restoring lung function. It includes oxygen therapy, aerosol therapy, physical therapy, and mechanical aids. All of these may be overused. One which has been questioned in recent years is intermittent positive pressure breathing (IPPB). A number of conferences and an extensive literature have not resolved many significant questions. It does seem clear that a simple device is as effective as an IPPB in delivering aerosol medication. Other indications have been criticized at least because of lack of data indicating benefit. No doubt because of this questioning, IPPB has been declining in use. In 43 Washington hospitals, the number of IPPB treatments per 100 admissions declined about 70 percent during the period 1976 to 1979. However, over the same period, other types of breathing aids (spirometry) and simple aerosol increased dramatically. This change is a move in the direction of less costly treatment modalities, which seems appropriate based on what is known about the efficacy of IPPB.

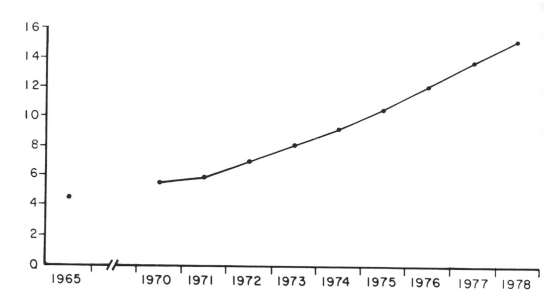

Figure 3. Cesarean section as a percentage of all deliveries in U.S. hospitals, by year

Data not available 1966-1969

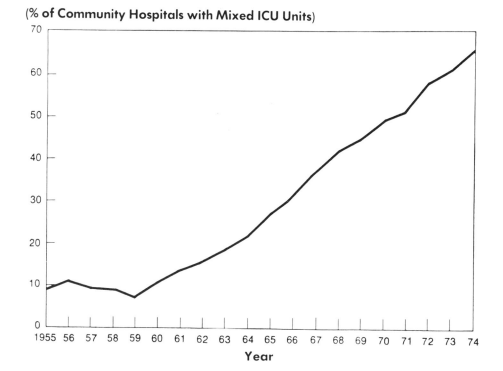

Figure 4. The diffusion of medical technologies: Intensive care units

Aphorism Six

Diagnostic technologies are probably used to considerable excess. However, their nature makes demonstration of this proposition difficult.

The field of diagnostic imaging is growing rapidly. In addition to conventional x-ray and CT scanning, it includes radionuclide scanning and ultrasound. The field of imaging now costs this country more than $10 billion a year. New technologies, such as nuclear magnetic resonance (NMR) and positron emission tomography (PETT), will complicate the picture further. Determining the value of any diagnostic test is difficult, compared to evaluating therapy. Most studies have dealt only with technical capability of a device or diagnostic accuracy. Few studies have examined the impact on therapy and virtually none have examined health outcome. Yet health outcome is the important factor. If making a diagnosis is the desirable outcome, then any added diagnostic test can be justified. However, examining health outcome is difficult, because that requires evaluating the therapy that follows the diagnosis and can take years.

Much the same argument can be made concerning clinical laboratory testing. There are now more than 700 tests provided in the clinical laboratory, many of them automated. Autoanalyzers can do 20 or more tests on one sample of blood. Many institutions have done a routine battery of tests to any patient on admission. Recently, insurance companies have changed their policies so as not to pay for routine testing.

A more specialized diagnostic procedure, cardiac radionuclide scanning, illustrates another aspect of this problem. Recent improvements in nuclear medicine technology have made it possible to image the coronary arteries. The technology is expanding very rapidly, with an estimated 227,000 procedures performed in 1978 with a cost of $100 million. Projected figures for 1981 are for 1.5 million scans and a cost of $425 million. The target population for cardiac imaging includes 12 million people in the United States with suspected or established coronary artery disease and an additional 80 million adults 40 years of age or older who might want to have a coronary artery screen. However, important questions remain about the value of this information to the individual. And there does not seem to be a natural limit to the number of scans below the 90 million people mentioned above. Without clear definition of goals of testing, this expensive procedure will certainly be overused.

Aphorism Seven

Many technologies are unquestionably efficacious, but also very costly.

The much-quoted example is the treatment of end-stage renal disease (ESRD). Patients must be treated with either dialysis or transplant. Approximately 48,000 people are now on long-term dialysis, with thousands more coming into the program every year. There were about 53,000 people in the federally-funded ESRD program in 1981. That number is expected to rise to 60,000 in 1984. Renal dialysis is unquestionably efficacious; without it, most people in the ESRD program would die. It is also expensive. The cost of a year of dialysis in a center is about $30,000. The national cost of the ESRD program is now more than $1 billion.

The artificial heart is an example of a technology that has been in development for years. Recent development has been slowed because of concerns about the ultimate cost. The totally implantable artificial heart has been under development with federal support since the early 1960s. The artificial heart could be life-saving for those with severe heart disease. Bunker has estimated that 152,000 patients a year are candidates. Costs for an artifical heart implant would be as high as $75,000, including around $14,000 for the device itself.

Finally, joint implants are examples of expensive technology that does not save lives, but improves mobility and removes pain. Joint implants are now commonly done in the hip and knee joints. About 10 percent of the U.S. population suffers from some form of arthritis, and an estimated 140,000 implantations of hip and knee joints were performed in 1976. Each implant costs an estimated $6,600 in direct costs initially. This technology is spreading rapidly, and is being applied to other joints, including finger joints. It obviously is difficult to judge if pain is severe enough to justify implantation of an artificial joint.

Aphorism Eight

Increasingly, medical technology offers a small marginal benefit with a large marginal cost.

This applies not only to new technologies, but to technologies being used beyond their original indication, in people not initially envisioned as recipients. Joint implant is an example. Originally it was used only in people with a non-functioning joint. Now it is used as a treatment for pain. Hip joint implants could almost become universal in the elderly. A surgeon has predicted that they will soon be used to <u>prevent</u> arthritis.

The intensive care unit is another example of an established technology being used more widely. (Figure 4). As late as 1958, only about 25 percent of community hospitals with 300 or more beds reported an intensive care unit. However, the development of new equipment for patients with heart conditions led to cardiac intensive care units beginning in 1962. Intensive care has continued to grow with the development of neonatal intensive care, obstetric intensive care, and so forth. The benefits of intensive care are not clear-cut. The literature on cardiac intensive care, for example, shows no clear benefit. At best, it appears that the benefits of widespread intensive care are fairly small.

Neonatal intensive care presents special problems. Evidence seems to show clearly that neonatal intensive care does save the lives of newborns, especially those of low birth weight. One side effect is that a certain number of serious handicaps result. It is estimated that 16,000 lives were saved with neonatal intensive care in 1978, with the result of 350 severely handicapped individuals who would have died in an earlier time. The costs range from $1,800 to over $40,000 per patient. Cost-effectiveness analyses have indicated that the cost of treating severe handicaps in the under 1,000 gram group exceeds the economic benefits of saving the lives of those who would have died in this group. Financial incentives for increased neonatal intensive care are apparently resulting in a reduction of facilities for primary newborn care. The result is the application of intensive care procedures to normal term infants, with a resulting minimal benefit at high cost.

Finally, a new technology characterized by limited benefit and high cost is bone marrow transplant for leukemia and aplastic anemia. The outlook for these patients is poor, and bone marrow transplant does improve survival. For example, with conventional therapy, essentially all of those with aplastic anemia are dead within a year. With bone marrow transplant, more than half survive a year, and more than 40 percent are still alive after three years. The cost of a treatment, however, is $67,772. The quality of life of those surviving is also rather poor, because of drug effects, and so forth. A cost-effectiveness ratio of $105,755 per life was calculated for bone marrow transplant for aplastic anemia, and a figure of $277,239 was estimated for acute leukemia. This is considerably more expensive than other life saving interventions.

Aphorism Nine

The system of payment for health care generously rewards the provision of new, machine-oriented technology and appears to inadequately reward more routine services, including counseling and prevention.

If the payment system were neutral, physicians would be paid about the same amount for a given amount of time whatever they were doing. There might be some differential fees to compensate for difficult and demanding tasks, longer time in training, etc. However, existing fees are very far from neutral.

Considering machine cost, maintenance, supplies, personnel, etc., it cost about $130 in 1976 to provide a CT scan. The fee for the scan averaged about $250. The fee of the radiologist is usually about $50. It generally takes about five to ten minutes to read a scan.

In contrast, a practitioner might collect a fee of $20 for a 15 minute office visit.

Upper gastrointestinal endoscopy is equally lucrative. The procedure takes about 15 minutes, and the average fee is about $240. It has been estimated that the cost of providing the procedure is about $40.

The new procedure radial keratotomy is even more striking. An ophthalmologist can do it in the office in about 15 minutes. The fee averages $1,500.

Aphorism Ten

Medical technology is associated with medical specialization, which itself is associated with costly health care. Controlling technology without attention to the numbers and mix of health manpower seems unlikely to control costs.

By 1976, only 39 percent of all active U.S. physicians were in primary care specialties of general and family practice, internal medicine, and pediatrics. Specialization has resulted in part from technology: radiology from x-ray, nuclear medicine from radioisotopes, vascular surgery from techniques including implantation of blood vessels and replacement of vessels with grafts. Residency positions in the new specialty are created to train physicians to use new technologies and to provide services to patients in hospitals that provide the new specialized services. But the presence of a cadre of specialists stimulates the use of their services. To earn their incomes, physicians pursue their practice, and in so doing attract sophisticated equipment and its accompanying manpower.

Medical education now depends on hospital-based clinical training dominated by a full-time faculty of specialists. Medical education entails the socialization of those entering the medical profession to that model. Students are oriented to rely on and to use the specialized technologies housed in a teaching hospital and to pursue specialty practice, with its higher prestige and income.

Greater specialization may follow from an excess supply of physicians. The supply of physicians is projected to rise from 450,000 in 1980 to 600,000 in 1990. The percentage of those in primary care is projected to rise only to 42 percent. As mentioned, prevailing payment methods make it possible to use specialized technologies to maintain income. Already the United States has a per capita rate of surgery considerably above that of such countries as Canada, in part because of our large number of surgeons per capita. The recently published report of the Graduate Medical Education National Advisory Committee (GMENAC) estimated surpluses in 1990 of such specialties as radiology, pathology, general surgery, orthopedic surgery, ophthalmology, and neurosurgery.

The country also has a substantial number of specialized health personnel other than physicians. Between 1970 and 1979, the number of people employed in the health service industry rose from about 4.2 million to about 6.8 million. The number of personnel per patient in community hospitals has risen from 302 per 100 patients in 1970 to 379 per 100 in 1978. Many of these personnel are trained to deal with the specialized technology of modern medical care.

Summary and Conclusions

These aphorisms have evolved out of studying the benefits, risks, and costs of specific medical technologies for
more than five years.

Are there any general lessons that emerge from these
cases?

The cases illustrate the era of chronic, life-threaten-
ing disease. The physician has an imperative to intervene,
and naturally, the patient wants the intervention if there
is hope of benefit, even if the cost is high. The cost to
the patient will usually be small because of the extent of
insurance. The fees reward physicians generously for providing technological services. Such forces as malpractice
also promote the use of technology.

Up to now, the main approach to managing technological
change and the costs of medical care has been regulatory.
The health planning program and the Professional Standards
Review Organization (PSRO) program are the main programs
used. This approach has obviously not been sufficient to
rationalize technology.

Other strategies, largely unexamined for their effect
on medical technology, are possible as an alternative to
regulation. Over the long term, changes in medical education could change the use of technology. Physicians could
be encouraged more vigorously to enter primary care specialties. They could also be trained more rigorously in evaluating benefits and costs of their technology.

Health maintenance organizations use technology differ-
ently from the health care system as a whole, and are able
to provide care more cheaply. With better information on the
effects of different organizations on technology, the types
of organizations that make more judicious decisions about
the adoption and use of technology could be supported. Of
course, this approach also means larger organizations in
health care, which could mean bureaucratization and dehu-
manization.

The last five years has brought technology assessment
or evaluation of the effects of technology prominence. It
appears that many technologies are overused, but good eval-
uative information is rarely available to show that defini-
tively. Physicians are motivated to provide good care to

their patients, and will respond, over time, to the results of evaluations. With the concern about costs in relation to benefits, formal studies such as cost-effectiveness analyses seem certain to be used more often in making policy decisions. A strategy to provide better information to practitioners should have positive effects.

However, none of these longer-term strategies can be expected to ameliorate the present situation unless there are also changes in the reimbursement system. In the short-run, the fee system seems likely to be used actively to channel technology. Fees can be set to discourage certain services or to encourage services. Reimbursement is already becoming contingent on the results of scientific evaluations of technology. Fees could be set at a level based on efficient use of technology. However, these piece-meal approaches do not seem likely to solve the problems identified in this paper. More sweeping reform of the insurance system seems likely, with such alternatives as capitation payment and prospective budgeting of hospitals growing in use.

There is another possibility, not in conflict with anything discussed in this paper, which needs to be considered. There are still unmet health needs in this country. There are worthwhile technologies not being fully applied. We are investing more than nine percent of our gross national product in health care expenditures, but who is to say that that is too much? As a society, we may choose to invest even more. My concern is not with how much we spend, but with how we spend that amount.

TECHNOLOGY ASSESSMENT
BY PHYSICIANS
Arnold S. Relman, M.D.

Is "technology," in fact, the major culprit behind the medical cost spiral? That depends on what is meant by the term. If one limited the definition to sophisticated devices like CT scanners and lasers and pacemakers and complex diagnostic and therapeutic procedures like coronary arteriography, hemodialysis, plasmapheresis, proton beam irradiation, and so on, then "technology" would be a significant but relatively small fraction of total health care costs. But in my opinion, that kind of definition, although widely used by some people, is inadequate because its boundaries are blurred. Where does "technology" stop being complex and sophisticated enough to qualify under this definition? One obviously cannot draw a sharp line anywhere. And when you think about it, if you know something about the practice of medicine, you come to the conclusion that it makes more sense to use a much broader and more comprehensive definition of medical "technology," such as: Any discrete and identifiable device, substance, procedure, or facility, used for the diagnosis, treatment, or prevention of disease.

That kind of definition was adopted by the Congress, for example, in the legislation that established the now defunct National Center for Health Care Technology. When this definition is used, the term "technology" can be applied to just about everything in medical practice--everything, that is, except the most important parts, i.e., history-taking, physical examination, clinical observation, decision-making and the counseling of patients. But my point is that, defined broadly, "technology" includes most of what is identified and billed as medical services to third parties, and it therefore accounts for most of the costs of health care. Hospitals, and all the special facilities and equipment they contain, also come under this definition. So the first conclusion I draw from a consideration of this subject is that technology assessment is virtually synonymous with the assessment of medical practice itself.

It follows from this conclusion that the regulatory approach, i.e., the governmental approach, to the assessment and evaluation of technology, amounts to nothing less than the regulation of medical practice. Therefore, my second conclusion is that the evaluation of technology, if it is to be done at all (and I hope to persuade you that it must be done more vigorously than ever before) should mainly be a responsibility of physicians. They will need help from others, but it is clearly up to them to provide professional leadership.

Much of medical practice as we know it today is untested or inadequately tested. So many new technologies are constantly being introduced that evaluation cannot keep up. We frequently introduce new techniques, new drugs, or new procedures into clinical practice on the basis of inadequate evidence. Even when the new technology has been heralded by some papers in the medical literature, the evidence is often deficient or lacking altogether. The literature describing a new test or technique may be little more than a collection of anecdotes or personal opinions. As a result, there is a progressive accumulation of medical procedures for which we have very little hard data about effectiveness (particularly in relation to other available technology), cost, or long-term safety.

Why should this be so? In the first place, it is very difficult to do proper, controlled clinical testing. It may in fact be impossible or unethical. It is often very expensive and it may take a long time. But there are other reasons that are not so understandable. There are other kinds of economic considerations, involving not just physicians, but the manufacturers and the purveyors of the devices and the techniques and the facilities. These self-serving economic considerations often play a powerful role. Some other factors are more justifiable and more defensible, it seems to me, and that is the natural tendency for physicians to want to do anything that might be of benefit to their patient, even if there is some doubt or uncertainty as to how effective the technique may be. If it might be of help, and if there is reasonable assurance that it will not make the patient worse, why not use the new technology? There is, in short, a strong tendency for doctors to want to be as helpful as they can and to use all the tools at their disposal.   And for the most part, there is a strong tendency among patients to want to have their doctors do just that.

Unfortunately, there is also a reluctance on the part of many physicians to put their clinical judgment to close scrutiny.   There is a tendency to feel that one's clinical judgment and experience, the last case that one saw, is enough basis to decide whether a particular clinical procedure is really helpful or not.   There is a general indisposition to expose oneself to the merciless judgment of the objective data derived from controlled studies.   And yet, when put to the test, the clinical impressions and personal opinions of even the most experienced and astute physicians are often proven wrong.   It is a painful and difficult lesson, for it is only human to want to feel confident about one's clinical decisions, particularly when patients need to depend on them.

I do not mean to imply that all unproven procedures are ineffective, but there are almost certainly many ineffective procedures among the numerous untested technologies now in use.   Many experienced clinicians believe (and I agree with them) that at least 10 or 20 percent of the diagnostic and therapeutic procedures carried out in the practice of medicine are either worthless or unnecessary or are being inappropriately and excessively used.   There are probably an equal percentage, another 10 or 20 percent, that are of questionable or borderline value--that are very close to the flat part of the cost-benefit curve.   The trouble is that we often cannot be sure which procedures are worthwhile and which are not, because we simply do not have the necessary information.   Despite the enormous effort expended by conscientious clinical investigators and clinicians all over the world to obtain new information, I am convinced that the gap is growing between what we do, and what we really know about what we do.   That does not mean that our power to diagnose and treat effectively is diminishing.   Obviously not; we are able to help our patients much more now than ever before.   But at the same time we are doing an increasing number of unproven or inadequately evaluated tests and procedures.

New drugs are evaluated by the Food and Drug Administration (FDA) for their safety and therapeutic efficacy, but to be approved by the FDA, a drug does not have to be compared with other drugs. Thus, new and expensive drugs may be introduced when there are already less costly ones available to do the same job, just as well or even better. Furthermore, once approved, a drug may be used in any way that a physician sees fit. Thus, despite the FDA, we have many drugs being used for purposes not evaluated by the FDA. The net result is that drugs are often used without sufficient evidence of effectiveness, or safety.

There is, of course, no FDA system for surgical operations, radiologic imaging techniques, endoscopy, sonography or for most medical procedures other than the use of drugs. For example, there is no mechanism to assure the evaluation of the effectiveness of hemodialysis or plasmapheresis, or inhalation therapy, or physiotherapy, or chiropractice manipulation, or dietotherapy or any of the many things that we physicians do all the time. And there is no FDA for the evaluation of laboratory tests. All of these, if they are to be evaluated at all, must be evaluated in the private sector with whatever resources are available.

Now obviously a lot of clinical evaluation goes on at present. I ought to know. Every year more than 3,000 new manuscripts are sent to the New England Journal of Medicine, many of which deal with the evaluation of new drugs, tests or procedures. But all the papers of this kind that are sent to all the medical journals in the world do not come close to doing the job. Many very important new and old modalities of diagnosis and treatment still remain unexamined or inadequately examined.

The fact of the matter is that not nearly enough money is being spent on the evaluation of medical technology. Two years ago, the National Institutes of Health (NIH) had a budget of over $3 billion, but only about $120 or $130 million of that was spent on the evaluation of clinical procedures, more than a third of which was being devoted to the evaluation of cancer chemotherapy. One major multi-institutional clinical trial of a new drug or treatment may cost $5 or $10 million, so $120 or $130 million will not buy very much in the way of clinical evaluation. The drug companies and the instrument manufacturers, of course, spend money on the development and assessment of the new drugs and new devices they hope to market, but this does not begin to meet the total need. The Congressional Office of Technology Assessment estimates that no more than $200 million are currently being spent by public agencies on the evaluation of medical technology in this country. At the same time government is spending over $100 billion to pay for the use of that technology.

The academic medical centers, where most of the work of technology evaluation should take place, have not done much to help this situation. Until now they have not acted as if they placed much value on this kind of clinical investigation. Even in those happy days when there was more money to support all kinds of clinical investigation and when it might have been possible to conduct more clinical evaluation studies, the best academic institutions were not very interested in the assessment of clinical procedures and tests. Basic laboratory research by clinical full-time faculty has always enjoyed higher standing in the academic medical community than applied clinical research. Papers published in good basic science journals or in the Journal of Clinical Investigation have carried greater weight with promotions committees than those in the best clinical journals. There is also the fact that clinical trials usually involve many people and many institutions, and individual rewards are limited. When many people are involved, the credit is diffused. And that is not very attractive to young faculty members who are interested in advancing their careers. Clinical trials also tend to be laborious and slow; they offer a relatively small yield of publishable papers for a relatively large expenditure of time and effort. It has generally been much easier to establish one's academic reputation by concentrating efforts on laboratory research, or at least on clinical studies of a more focused and basic character.

But now the need for clinical trials and more assessment of medical technology has become more pressing than ever, and it is time for a broad national program. The establishment of the National Center for Health Care Technology a few years ago seemed to portend the development of such a program, but the Center never got off the ground. Its maximum funding was about $4 million and it lasted only a few years before it was "zeroed out" of the Reagan administration's budget. The Center is gone now and there is nothing in government to take its place. In my judgment, that was a very unwise and costly decision for the administration, because the Center had the potential of saving the government a lot of money now being wasted on unnecessary and ineffective--but unidentified--medical technology.

Of course, we have had a program of Consensus Devel-

opment Conferences at the NIH, and we have the new Clinical Efficacy Assessment Project (CEAP) by the American
College of Physicians. We also have a statement by the
American Medical Association that it will undertake some
assessment of medical technology. These programs and plans
are admirable and can make useful contributions, but we
need new information about technology much more than
simply a consensus by a committee of experts based on
current inadequate data. We need new clinical studies, and
new data--and you cannot generate those by sitting around a
committee table.

What kind of new data are needed? First of all, we require many more randomized controlled clinical trials. But
they are not the only, and sometimes not even the best, way
to find out about medical procedures. We can use epidemiologic techniques, where one simply studies statistical asso-
ciations, without carrying out any experimental intervention.
One can employ various kinds of statistical methods to look
at relations between phenomena, either retrospectively or
prospectively, and sometimes this yields very useful data.
One can also simply collect and organize clinical data in data
banks, using new computerized techniques of data storage
and retrieval. With the use of the computer, we can store
information about clinical experience so that we do not have
to depend on anyone's memory or clinical impressions, and
we can accumulate a total experience far beyond anything
that could be acquired by one person or one institution. In
situations where it is unethical or impractical to conduct a
trial, or where control observations are not possible, this
kind of data accumulation can be very useful in the evaluation of medical technology. And then, finally, we can do
cost-effectiveness studies in which information about effectiveness of technology is related to costs, and we thereby
arrive at a picture of how much benefit we get for how much
cost.

We need all of these kinds of information, and more, if
we are going to do a proper job of assessing our health care
technology. How can such a program be funded? Some time
ago I made a proposal in an editorial in the New England
Journal of Medicine, which I offer again here. I suggest
that all of the third-party payers in this country, including the "Blues," the private insurance companies, and HCFA
(all of the agencies that pay for the costs of medical care)
agree to contribute a very small fraction of the total
amount of money they pay for medical care to a central fund
for technology evaluation. If that fraction were 0.2 of one

percent a year, it would amount to something of the order of $400 or $500 million. Such a fund could be used to support a private agency that would give competitive grants and contracts for assessment studies of all kinds. I share the widely expressed view that the evaluation of medical practice should be conducted by the private sector on a voluntary basis. The agency thus established would not only be responsible for subsidizing research but also for gathering and disseminating information. As a private agency, it should not have responsibility for deciding which procedures are to be reimbursed and which are not. It should have no regulatory authority. It should not be telling doctors how to practice medicine or what is good medicine. It should simply be a non-profit public service that helps physicians to find out what they need to know about the use of medical technology by underwriting the costs of the necessary studies.

Medical journals must play a major role by facilitating the publication of useful, critically reviewed papers on technology assessment. Medical schools and research institutions must encourage interest in evaluation, and should reward faculty who do it well, with academic appointments and promotion. The schools should teach decision analysis and evaluation techniques and should do whatever they can to increase awareness of the need for more critical assessment of health care practices. Those responsible for graduate medical education also have a major responsibility in this endeavor.

Let physicians decide how to use the new information generated by such a program. Skeptics will wonder whether the availability of information will by itself be sufficient to modify the behavior of physicians. That remains to be seen, but I confidently predict that it will. In my opinion, doctors are more interested in practicing good medicine and in being perceived by their colleagues as being good doctors, than they are in anything else. I believe that a doctor's pride in doing his job well and his concern for taking good care of patients will help to moderate the other perverse economic incentives that now influence the use of medical technology. So, I think that doctors will respond to clear, new information about technology by modifying their behavior in whatever ways that are appropriately responsive to the facts. They always have done so in the past and I see no reason to doubt that they will continue to do so--provided that the new information is convincing and commands the support of the experts.

I am not suggesting that every study which this new agency sponsors would yield decisive, clean-cut results. Obviously that will not be the case, nor will the experts often agree. But we have dealt with that kind of situation all along. We know that we do not always get clear answers, but every good study we do, and every investment we make in good science, pays off sooner or later in more understanding and in improvement of our practice of medicine. The payoff here would be in terms of a vastly enhanced understanding of which medical procedures work, and which do not; which are cost-effective, and which are not. This understanding would inevitably lead to a more discriminating employment of medical technology, the abandonment of useless or unnecessary procedures, and a more economical and effective use of medical resources.

Of course, we must at the same time deal with the countervailing economic forces that encourage excessive, uncritical use of technology by physicians. Our fee structure needs overhauling. We have too many specialists, and probably we are now producing too many physicians, and these problems must also be dealt with in some sensible way. I have also written and said many times that I think that doctors, in order to preserve their professional integrity and their standing before the public, will have to separate themselves from any entrepreneurial involvement in health care businesses. To be trusted as the advocate of the public interest, practicing physicians should limit their financial involvement in health care to the income they derive directly from their personal professional services.

Summary

I take a somewhat different view of the present dilemma about the control of health care costs. This subject is usually discussed in terms of two options: (1) we have more federal regulation--more legislation, more heavy-handed, bureaucratic, inefficient control of medical practice--or (2) we depend on the marketplace and we let price competition decide on the allocation of services. I do not believe that either of those solutions is very good. For many reasons, I have serious reservations about relying on a competitive marketplace for the distribution of health care. I am not persuaded that the marketplace would preserve the quality of services, freedom of choice by physicians and patients, equity, access, and all the things that we consider to be important in the delivery of health care.

There is a third option: Put the responsibility for controlling costs and maintaining quality clearly in the hands of the medical profession and give it help by supporting a national program of health care evaluation, along with other reforms in the education and reimbursement of physicians. Our physicians are the key. We should work on changing what physicians do voluntarily, before we consider changing the system in any more radical way, or before we try any more regulation. It is much better to improve the way physicians use technology than to limit the development of new technology with regulations or to do anything that would slow the introduction and diffusion of new ideas. On the other hand, allowing the development and utilization of new technology to proceed on its present course will lead to unsupportable costs and an irresistible call for more regulation.

The medical profession holds the key to this dilemma, but it needs more and better information before it can take any action. A modest investment by the third parties in providing a system of technology assessment would provide large payoffs in terms of a more efficient use of technology and a generally higher quality of care. There are not many policies that can realistically be expected to help control costs while improving the quality of care. Expanded technology assessment under the kind of program I have described offers that kind of promise.

PHYSICIAN REMUNERATION: BOONDOGGLE OR BUST?
Benson B. Roe, M.D.

Generalities About Remuneration

Factors that determine what people get paid for their efforts and talents are obviously complex. In a free market economy the price of any product or service becomes the level at which the demand just keeps the marginal producer in business. Scarcity, quality and the economic productivity of the item all tend to raise prices. Whereas competition and abundant supply tend to keep prices down. In a controlled or socialistic economy, on the other hand, these factors are distorted or superceded by political pressures to provide artificial price supports and subsidies. Rate controls may be imposed to keep prices below what might be paid in a market of scarcity. More often, however, these so-called controls keep prices elevated beyond what would be sustained in free competition. The extent to which the consumer/taxpayer should be expected to underwrite above-market prices for the sake of society's broad interests is a matter of endless debate.

Since I am not an economist, it behooves me not to dwell on the morality and justification for paying a professional athlete a million dollars a year and a school teacher a mere $16,000. It is important to stress, however, that athletes were low on the pay scale in the days when their remuneration derived only from gate receipts; whereas now they are performers that attract huge national audiences to watch television commercials fetching $300,000 to $800,000 a minute. Thus the "kitty" on which they can potentially draw is enormous and if their employers want them badly enough, the resources to pay well are available.

111

Basic Changes in Physician Remuneration

So it was with physicians who made their living out of the pockets of their patients--few of whom were wealthy. Most doctors practiced with little regard for remuneration; commonly their fees would slide according to the patient's ability to pay. Physicians collected what they could--which often turned out to be nothing. As a result doctors tended to be comfortable middle income earners. High income physicians were either those who did an enormous volume of work or who possessed a unique talent for which there was a large demand or who catered to a select group of wealthy patients. Realistically the average physician's "usual" fee was what he <u>hoped</u> to collect but usually did so only from the affluent or from those with multiple insurance policies.

When the government and the insurance industry came along with lots of megabucks to pay for medical care, the patient was essentially removed from the financial process. Organized medicine, that once had vigorously opposed Medicare, cleverly arranged (and had written into law) a system of reimbursement that virtually mandated issuing blank checks to providers, including physicians, hospitals and ancillary services. This is the UCR (Usual, Customary or Reasonable) system of payment which was predicated on "paying the going price" but instead turned out to be "paying whatever is charged." Predictably charges escalated very rapidly, first because the kitty was huge and was infinitely expandable through taxation and increased premiums, second because there were no built in constraints--the system was open ended, and third because there was no competitive element involved in the pricing process. At first this system seemed to be the best of all worlds for everyone concerned; the providers set their own prices and were guaranteed a comfortable profit; the patients got almost everything taken care of without having to reach into their pockets; and the whole process was maintained painlessly by employer supported insurance premiums or payroll-deducted taxes. Anyhow it did not matter how much it cost. America is a wealthy nation and political rhetoric declared that the best is none too good for the American people!

Background

It is important to recall the status of medical economics in the era prior to third-party involvement, essentially up to World War II, and to outline the course of events which emerged with the advent of Medicare, Medicaid, and almost universal health insurance shared by employers. Hospitals, for the most part were operated as charitable institutions; many were largely supported by endowments and all were heavily dependent on volunteer help in staffing and management. Wages were at the bottom of the scale and technology was infinitesimal by modern standards. When I returned from World War II the ward bed rates at the Massachusetts General Hospital had risen from $4.50 to $7.00 a day and the most expensive room in the private pavilion was something like a shocking $20. Certainly general inflation does not alone account for the current rates of $300 a day and $1000 a day for intensive care. Many factors are involved in the metamorphosis. Mushrooming competition for the diminishing charity dollar left hospitals with inadequate support from their traditional source. Unionization of hospital employees resulted in much higher wages for larger staffs who did less work. Hospital administration burgeoned from a couple of tiny offices to more than a whole floor containing a small batallion of salaried executive personnel with an army of paper shuffling secretaries. Although it can be argued that these changes corrected important deficiencies and reflected a growing technology, I can personally verify that the quality of patient care, the alleviation of suffering and the prolongation of life are only slightly improved today over what they were 30 years ago--the differences are infinitesimal by comparison with the escalation of cost.

Consequences of the New System

This new method of reimbursement (UCR) altered how and what medicine is practiced. Tests and procedures are compensated at a higher rate than pure professional time; thus office practice has been garnished with income-producing machinery. Hospitals have added many new services and facilities for which extra charges can be made, and even surgeons use gimmicks to compound a simple operation or to make it sound difficult.

The system has also led to misdirecting medical manpower both geographically and into specialties that are already heavily oversupplied. In several specialties the level of remuneration has become so high that a surgeon who does only an occasional case or who utilizes only a fraction of his capability by serving principally as an assistant, is able to gross over $100,000 a year. Consequently there is no incentive for the marginal and underutilized surgeon to move away from his chosen location to an area where his services are needed or to provide some other aspect of medical care that may be in greater demand.   Thus the absence of competitive forces in the system offers an incentive to inflate prices, to overutilize the more remunerative services, and to discourage physicians from providing other needed services.   Under the current system, ironically, an oversupply of specialists in an area does NOT drive prices <u>down</u> from competition but rather forces them <u>up</u> to levels that will comfortably support the underworked.

Abuses of the New System

Because the third party is in effect mandated to pay virtually all charges and because the system lacks controls, it has literally <u>invited</u> abuse.   Some of the abuses reflect outright fraud which the nature of the system has merely facilitated and made difficult to stop.   Some of the abuses could be described as no worse than generous interpretations of loose definitions.   In certain instances these questionable practices are rationalized as justifiable attempts to correct inequities in the system (the underpaid physician who charges for office lab work).   And most of the offenders are simply going along with the crowd.   Who can be blamed for billing what lesser physicians are collecting, particularly if it is not coming out of the patient's pocket?

The extent of these abuses is suggested by the results of my personal survey of cardiac surgical claims to California Blue Shield in 1979-80 when Blue Shield paid out more money, by some 20 percent, for coronary bypass operations than for any other surgical procedure.   Blue Shield's average pay-out at that time--to the surgeon alone--was $3,500 to $4,200 per uncomplicated case, and I recently learned that the Southern California billing average this year has risen to $6,500.   This fee, which I consider to be preposterous, does <u>not</u> include--and is supplemented by--charges for usually two assistants currently at $1,200 apiece, anesthesia at $1,500, plus substantial fees for cardiologists and intensive care physicians who conduct much of the post-operative management.   If these fees were to be applied country-wide for approximately 125,000 coronary bypass operations in 1981 and added to the hospital costs (averaging $20,000 in Los Angeles), a price tag of $3.5 billion could be projected. This expenditure would provide largely symptomatic (non-curative) help for only 0.05 percent of the U.S. population.

A 1979 survey determined that essentially all of these

operations were being performed by about 700 surgeons, which would average out to a comfortable four cases per week. Assuming a "modest" fee of $3,000, which is less than half the Southern California average, these surgeons will derive an annual income of over half a million dollars a year. That conservative estimate is for the <u>average</u> income from <u>one</u> operation; it does not include the other cardiac and thoracic operations these surgeons perform nor does it reflect the income of the moderately busy surgeon who easily performs 10 or more coronary bypass operations a week.

The early days of cardiac surgery were characterized by blood, sweat and tears; each case was a dramatic effort, involving innovation, uncertainty and long hours. The surgeon participated in the diagnostic studies and preoperative preparation, planned and directed technical details of the extracorporeal circulation, conducted the entire long operation, and personally supervised every detail of postoperative management, often spending late nights at the bedside. High fees were perhaps warranted in those days. But today things are different. Cardiac surgery is provided on a huge scale with automated routines; improved methods and accumulated experience have provided safety and seeming simplicity. Two or three open-heart cases a day are now common for many cardiac surgeons and some do even more. This increased capacity is feasible because the surgeon's global responsibilities are now far less challenging and because many of those responsibilities have been delegated to other professionals. Cardiologists now provide reliable diagnostic details and prepare the patient for operation; anesthesiologists expertly provide physiological stability, allowing the surgeon to come and go with minimal concern; pump technicians have assumed professional expertise in the operation of heart-lung machines as reliably as water comes out of the tap; standardized techniques have shortened the operating time and minimized complications; and a separate team effectively administers postoperative care. Each of these services, of course, is now billed separately over and above the surgical fee. Under these circumstances it would be expected that the surgeon's fee would have dropped as his unit capacity increased, but instead of dropping the fee has multiplied five or six times.

Admittedly this scenario represents one of the worst offenders (cardiac surgeons) and one of the worst areas (California), but it is by no means unique. Neurosurgeons, plastic surgeons, ophthalmologists, orthopedists, and urologists are in the same category and the rest of medical care is not far behind. And there is nothing to prevent this pattern from spreading throughout medicine.

For centuries the medical profession has attracted honorable and conscientious people. The ethical code of physicians promoted a sense of dedication and "nobility" that superceded monetary gain. This heritage probably at least slowed down the course of economic devastation that the system has now wrought. But large amounts of money, easily gained, tend to have a pernicious effect on how people behave. I fear that physicians are trampling their benevolent image in a stampede to the pot of gold.

Addressing the Problem

That a serious problem exists is not in dispute. The health care cost for this year will exceed the defense budget and by the end of the decade it is expected to exceed $900 billion or $3,000 per man, woman and child.

Solutions to the problem are not clearly evident--except to those of a socialistic mind who would point out that we are the only industrialized country in the world without socialized medicine and that the present shambles justifies such a course. History has demonstrated the pitfalls of that pathway, and I hope it will not occur. But unless the profession shoulders its responsibility and works with the insurance industry to provide a financially viable system of health financing, I am not optimistic about the future.

The patient/consumer--under the present system--does not represent the marketplace because he has no capacity to judge cost effectiveness, no information to determine competitive pricing, and little or no direct financial responsibility for paying the bill. The real consumer is the third party carrier who supposedly acts as an agent for the patient, though perhaps not always protecting the patient's economic interests, and who dispenses the money that supports the whole technology. Ultimately, of course, the public does pay the cost through insurance premiums or taxation. Until recently those burdens have been tolerable and the realities were obscured in the fringe of labor costs and government services. But the problem has now escalated to major proportions that impact everyone. It is now a monster, gulping significant hunks of the average man's income. The cost of health care is no longer ignored by the public as a peripheral issue. The growing attention given to the subject by the media both reflects and compounds public awareness of the problem. To address it with rhetoric or to respond with less than effective remedies is certain to be disastrous.

Curbing these trends may be nearly impossible in the presence of a firmly entrenched social philosophy that declares all-out first class medical care to be a basic human right, and a traditional medical philosophy that espouses the unrestricted use of heroic measures even against ridiculous odds. In my opinion we will eventually have to face up to triage in civilian medicine because highly sophisticated, enormously expensive life-support mechanisms are in the wings that could sustain some semblance of life almost indefinitely. But that is another subject.

The economic monster simply <u>must</u> be curbed. Health care is inherently expensive and it is bound to become more so. If society is to afford it and if the bulk of the population is to benefit from it, this care has <u>got</u> to be delivered more efficiently, more selectively and at a more reasonable cost. Inevitably this means that everything cannot be done for everybody, that redundant and underutilized facilities and personnel must be phased out, and that the public subsidy must be limited to basic pricing and not luxury pricing.

Open Competition

One proposal has been to allow market forces to operate with open advertising and competitive pricing. This mechanism would undoubtedly reduce costs, but it is doubtful that our society would tolerate the consequences of bankrupting thousands of inefficient or low occupancy hospitals and starving out thousands of the underutilized oversupply of physicians who are currently surviving--and even thriving--on current astronomical fees. Such a system would create many local imbalances and inequities which might be tolerated in the beer and soap market but would almost certainly disrupt the humanitarian objectives of health care. Furthermore, its implementation would require the patient/customer to have a financial stake in the payment process, which is contrary to the desire for "full coverage."

Negotiated Reimbursement Scales

My own proposal is to replace the major culprit, the UCR system, with a fixed reimbursement scale subject to periodic revision which would be negotiated with each specialty group through its responsible leaders. To be eligible for reimbursement a physician would have to agree to accept the established amount as payment in full for all patients covered by Medicare, Medicaid, and certain labor-contract policies. Under other policies he would be permitted to apply additional charges to patients, providing the patient is informed of any surcharge <u>before</u> the service is rendered and provided patients are educated to the fact that competent services are available without a surcharge. Such an arrangement would not restrict what any physician can <u>charge</u> in his private practice, only what he will <u>get</u> from the third party. Administrative costs and fraudulent claims could be materially reduced by defining the coverage comprehensively to include compounded problems, management of complications and support of ancillary personnel. Obliterating supplemental payments for these "extras" would provide incentive against unnecessary utilization and would indirectly reward the physician with the least complicated and most expeditious results--which is the opposite of the present system.

Counterarguments

It will be argued that this proposal is nothing but a reversion to the old indemnification system which was abandoned because people wanted complete coverage and found themselves stuck for too many extras. The difference, however, is that surcharging (except where specifically permitted) will disqualify the physician from any subsequent reimbursement from the carrier.

Much, of course, will be made of the "free choice" issue. But realistically this is nonsense. In almost four decades of practice I have seen only a half dozen patients that showed even the slightest hesitation about accepting a referral recommendation or that made suggestions of their own; most patients go willingly to whatever hospital and to whatever consultant they are sent. Anyhow the system I have proposed will undoubtedly provide several options in every field. I support the belief that patients should have choices and not be forced to accept a physician whom they dislike or distrust. But there is no justification for these choices to include unreasonable and exorbitant costs.

Proponents of unrestricted free choice contend that the economically disadvantaged would be deprived of the "best" physicians, erroneously assuming that fees were proportional with skill and experience. My own review of California Blue Shield payments reveals this assumption not only to be false but actually to be the opposite of reality.   The well-established and best-known surgeons generally had modest charges, whereas the highest charges were made by those most recently in practice, possibly because they had no previous "profile" which they were obliged to follow or because they had so few patients that they could not survive without high fees.

Those who will resist returning to a fixed reimbursement system will need to be reminded that agencies, such as the Crippled Children's Service, have operated successfully on that basis for nearly 35 years, and the quality of their physician panels has been of the highest order.

I am certain that any proposal to change the status quo can and will be criticized.   Change will not be easy because much of our present system is cast in concrete--in the form of contracts, laws, and agency regulations.   Whatever we do is bound to be imperfect.   But unless we do it--unless we restore fiscal integrity to medical economics--the whole dream of independent American Medicine will turn into a pumpkin!

MONITORING MEDICAL TECHNOLOGY: SHALL TECHNOLOGY BE REGULATED? HOW AND BY WHOM?
Ruth S. Hanft

Although my topic for discussion is regulation of technology, my own position falls between a laissez faire approach to technology and a direct regulatory approach. I do not believe that market forces and competition alone, without a systematic mechanism for assessing technology and disseminating the findings, will resolve problems of use, distribution and cost inflation. I also do not believe that regulatory approaches such as certificate of need or rate regulation can be rational and effective without such assessments. An organized monitoring and assessment process is necessary.

The reason for discussing the impact of technology is the recognition that the increasing costs of health care are in large part attributable to technology and its diffusion. In an era of resource constraints, these increased costs preclude the use of national resources for other social purposes. The report of the Subcommittee on Health and the Environment which accompanied the bill establishing the National Center for Health Care Technology noted:

"There is an emerging consensus...that many technologies have been widely adopted into medical practice in the face of disturbingly scanty information about their health benefits, clinical risks, cost effectiveness and social side effects. In addition, the use of some technologies persists long after it becomes evident that these technologies are of marginal utility, outmoded and even harmful." 1/

Some specific examples that stimulated Congressional

action and this Norfleet Forum are the following:

o   Expenditures for coronary bypass surgery are $2 billion a year.

o   A heart transplant costs a minimum of $100,000 per procedure and requires maintenance care of about $10,000 per year. About 50 procedures are done each year and it is estimated that this number could grow to 2,000 to 4,000 per year.

o   Renal dialysis costs the economy $1 billion and is rapidly rising toward $2 billion.

o   Cesarean section deliveries in some hospitals now account for 20 percent of all births at a cost of about twice a normal delivery.

o   Plasmapheresis for arthritis, a procedure not proven effective, costs about $40,000 in the first year of treatment, and is diffusing rapidly with the establishment of plasmapharesis centers similar to dialysis centers.

o   A stay in a neonatal intensive care unit averages $30,000 for infants below 1000 grams. Many of these infants do not survive and many have neurological and other disabling illnesses.

o   Medicare spends 20 percent of its funds for people in their last year of life and 80 percent of its funds for 20 percent of the Medicare population.

o   The fastest growing sector of population is the elderly, who consume 2.5 to 3 times the amount of services as those under 65 years of age.

o   At the current inflation rate national health expenditures are projected to consume 12 percent of the gross national product by 1990.

o   Intensity of services or technology accounts for about one third of the increase in health care expenditures.

In an era of finite resources, it is clear that rising consumption of health services affects society's ability to meet other demands and needs, whether in the domestic or the defense sectors of the economy.

During the past 10 years consciousness about the impact of new technology has risen, as evidenced by numerous conferences like this on the impact of technology; development of research in technology assessment at universities and other research centers, and by specialty societies; studies of ethical issues related to technology; consensus conferences at the National Institutes of Health (NIH); the development of the Office of Technology Assessment of the Congress; the enactment of the medical device legislation; and the development of the National Center for Health Care Technology (NCHCT).

It is not that advances in medical science--prolongation of life, reduction of disability and pain--are not deemed highly desirable.   Rather, the issues are the effectiveness of the technology; the appropriateness of its use; the diffusion of the technology and its pricing; the ethical issues inherent in the distribution of goods and services given finite resources; and who shall decide who gets what.

History of Technology Assessment

Technology assessment is not new to society and certainly not new to the medical community. Such assessments, although not necessarily systematic, are a normal part of the decision making of practitioners as well as a major aspect of the development of new drugs, devices, modes of care.   Indeed, the history of modern medicine is the story of the development and testing of medical technology. The basic diagnostic tools of modern medicine--the stethoscope, the clinical laboratory, x-rays--symbolize more than simple feats of technological development; they stand as watersheds in medical knowledge, for each of these technologies embodied a new way of perceiving the body and its diseases.

As physicians applied the developing scientific and technologic insights of allied fields to the diagnosis and treatment of disease, they devised more effective devices and techniques. This century has seen the most rapid development of medical innovation. Since the 1930s, when the armamentarium of the physician was limited, there has been a literal explosion of technology.   To cite a few: sulfa drugs, antibiotics, chemotherapy, lasers, organ transplantation, CT scans, nuclear imaging. The current breakthroughs in genetics-DNA engineering may well make other recent advances pale by comparison. The development of technologies was incremental, with refinement through evaluation, experiment and redevelopment. That process, continuing today, is of fundamental importance.

The advances in technology since World War II have had numerous consequences, not limited to the substantial improvement in health status. For example, the complexity of technology is reflected in the extended residencies and fellowships physicians pursue; the development of a host of allied health professionals needed to man complex technology, who seek and achieve credentials and licenses; increases in the number of personnel per hospital bed; increased services per visit or per hospital stay; and pricing of new services at higher rates than older treatment patterns. The rapid advances in technology have also raised substantial moral issues concerned with definitions of death, human experimentation, and the right to live and the right to die.

Regulation in Health Care--Types of Regulation

With the current negative political reaction to regulation, the concept of systematic technology assessment as embodied in the legislation creating the National Center for Health Care has been subsumed in anti-regulation debates and activities.

Regulation in health care, primarily peer regulation by the healing professions and religious behavioral codes related to health, are ancient traditions. Both the Hippocratic and Maimonidean oaths are a form of regulation; a code of ethics. Genesis, the Talmud and its commentaries, and the Koran list behavioral and dietary admonitions that probably can be attributed to early public health concerns. During the Middle Ages quarantine regulations were established to halt the spread of plagues and this type of regulation continues to the present time.

Today regulation has a negative connotation, yet it is important to distinguish the different types of "regulation" by purpose and process. Regulation in health care has been driven primarily by the concepts of the protection of human life, the injunction in the medical code to "do no harm" and, more recently, the concept of the "quality of care." Regulation in health care, contrary to current rhetoric, did not spring forth with Medicare and Medicaid and the social programs of the sixties. Medicare, in fact, adopted existing private regulatory processes such as the Joint Commission on the Accreditation of Hospitals, licensure, etc. Even today, programs like Professional Standards Review are controlled and implemented by the private sector.

Until the 1940s there were two main streams of regulation in health: public regulation addressed to societal public health issues--quarantine, disease control and surveillance for communicable disease, protection of water, air, food, drugs and sanitation; and regulation by the profession to assure quality of care. While in today's environment questions have been raised as to the extent, complexity and costs of "public health" regulation, few question the role of regulation in public health. The regulation of health care services is still primarily private regulation by the professions themselves, enforced by state licensure bodies composed largely of members of the profession. To put the regulation debate in perspective, let me cite some of the private sector regulatory activities which may be enforced or reinforced by government, but which are privately initiated and operated. These include accreditation, certification and licensure of educational facilities, programs and professions; professional practice acts; accreditation of hospitals; professional disciplinary activities; and hospital admitting privileges.

A third stream of regulation is more recent than public health regulation or professional regulation and began with the advent of private third party payments and accelerated after World War II with the growth of insurance. The decision to pay or not to pay and to whom is an implicit form of regulation. When a third party deems a service payable on an inpatient basis and not on an outpatient basis, the third party is regulating the use of services and the site of services. This third regulatory stream has grown in importance as Medicare and Medicaid adopted private systems of accreditation, definitions of covered services, and enforced the standards through payment or non-payment of services.

Medicare also adopted the private insurance concept of "medically necessary services" or "reasonable and necessary" services. Until recently, this concept was ill defined and decisions in the public and private sector were made on an ad hoc, decentralized basis, usually through consultation with the medical advisor of an insurance company or through consultation with specialty societies.

Medical Decision Making--Costs, Ethics, Technology

Innovation in health care technology continues to present a number of problems. The efficacy and safety of a technology is not always apparent at an early stage. Clinical trials, for example, take a number of years before they provide sufficient information. Medical side effects of a technology, i.e., radiation for tonsillitis, resulting in a high incidence of thyroid cancer, or DES effects may not be apparent for 20 years.

Medical science is not a precise science--there are always grey areas where equally competent physicians, faced with similar diagnostic findings will choose different solutions. For example, a number of studies have shown wide variations in use of different surgical procedures in similar population groups. The NIH Consensus Conference on Cesarean section indicated a large variation in Cesarean intervention for "dystocia" and the NCHCT coronary bypass conference indicated wide variation patterns of diagnostic testing.

In addition, it is also difficult to link changes in health status to a particular technology or innovation. Is the decline in deaths from cardiovascular illness due to coronary care units, coronary bypass surgery--expensive technologies--or hypertension screening, changes in diet and cigarette smoking--inexpensive technologies? Or is it some combination of these, or a yet unknown factor? Is the decline in infant mortality attributable to advances in neonatal care, Cesarean section, improved utilization of prenatal care, better nutrition because of food stamps, the WIC program, higher education levels?

Then there are the complex ethical issues related to individual technologies and societal allocation of resources. Maternal serum alpha feto protein (MSAFP) is an example of such a complex issue. The test, proven effective by the Food and Drug Administration (FDA), screens for the congenital anomalies spinabifida and anencephaly. About half the children born with such defects do not survive beyond 24 hours of birth. Of those who survive, 75 percent will have serious physical and/or mental defects.

The screening test and its interpretation, however, present a number of problems and need to be followed by ultrasound diagnosis and amniocentesis. While the MSAFP test is inexpensive, the follow-up testing essential for a more definitive diagnosis is expensive. There is a short period of only two weeks in which the sequence of tests and appropriate genetic counseling must be received. Social issues related to the test include the potential for aborting normal fetuses if the sequence of tests is not undertaken, the availability and accessibility of amniocentesis and genetic counseling, and of course, payment for abortion if the fetus is affected and the family chooses to terminate the pregnancy.

Under current law, the MSAFP test falls under the FDA device provisions and the only issue for the FDA, which is the only regulatory agency involved, is the safety and efficacy of the testing reagent. Yet the release of the reagent, with no restrictions on use and follow up, precipitated numerous social issues related to the availability of a useful test, protection of the consumer and fetus from the possibility of an unnecessary abortion resulting from incomplete information, and the volatile issue of abortion itself.

Societal side effects, in terms of the use of scarce resources, may outweigh the benefits of a technology. In the case of heart transplants, the Massachusetts General Hospital decided not to develop a heart transplant capability, primarily because the resources consumed in capital and manpower would preclude the hospital from providing other valuable services; yet other institutions have made exactly the opposite decision.

How then should society handle these issues, assuming that society has concluded that some controls are needed on the proportion of the gross national product spent for health?

Most observers concede that the health industry is unique in its operations and, although greater market forces than are at work at present should and could be stimulated, health care is not and cannot be a traditional economic market. The life, death, and disability consequences of many medical decisions limit society's ability to question them and even to participate fully in the decision making, at the patient-physician micro-level. The physician, to a greater or lessor extent, acts as agent for the patient, deciding the range and scope of services to be provided. The ethos of the physician is to consider his patient's welfare first and to do all he can to save life and reduce morbidity, disability and pain. These cumulative micro-decisions exert a major impact on the cost of care. The combination of the lack of precision in medical decision making and the concern for the individual patient drives the decision making toward providing more rather than less. Compounding these factors are our methods of financing. In the case of inpatient hospital care, costs are paid for almost entirely by third parties, placing no immediate economic burden on the physician or patient. In the case of diagnostic tests, the patient is often fully insured for the service and the physician receives a fee for each individual test. Compounding these factors further is the fee structure which rewards technology-intensive services at higher rates than primary care services. And, finally, in health care, unlike other markets, the price of a technologic procedure does not always decline as it becomes more widely diffused. In many industries, new technology leads to greater efficiency, increased output and conserved resources, particularly manpower. Sophisticated technology in health care has led to a need for greater and more skilled manpower--further specialization. In health care, also, the more specialized new manpower often seeks the economic protection of credentialing and licensure, leading to less flexibility in the use of manpower.

Efforts have been made to affect costs through a number of regulatory devices such as more rational resource allocation by health planning; reviews of the use of services; and various rate regulation devices ranging from the economic stabilization program to state rate regulation and limits on Medicare payments to hospitals for drugs and now laboratory procedures. We are, however, an impatient nation and never seem to wait for the results of actions before we react, assuming failure.

Today the conceptual thrust is toward deregulation and the creation of a competitive market rather than regulation of costs or supply. Competition is the byword. However, few of the proposals to date remove the barriers to a market, or address the impact of an improved market on technology and its diffusion.

Monitoring Medical Technology

The rapid proliferation of medical technology and its perceived role in increasing health care costs has led to two major efforts--planning and reimbursement control--in the governmental and private sectors to place constraints on the introduction, distribution, and appropriateness of use of the technologies.

Health planning and certificate of need, which were designed primarily to address quantity and distribution issues, in their short life time have had an uneven but constraining effect on capital expansion of beds, hospital equipment and certain services. One of the major drawbacks in implementing these programs has been the lack of systematic information on specific technologies, need, and use rates. Obviously, this program, which is slated for termination by the Reagan administration, will have little future impact in most areas of the country.

Reimbursement constraints have taken three forms--professional standards review, rate regulation, and determinations of medical necessity. Professional standards review placed responsibility on local physicians' groups to review the appropriateness of care, particularly through review of hospital admissions and length of stay. In only a few localities have Professional Standards Review Organizations (PSROs) looked at technology, mainly at surgical rates and laboratory tests. The effect of the PSRO program is controversial, its decision making was highly decentralized, and its future support is unlikely.

Rate regulation is a program operated by a few states and seeks to put a ceiling on hospital costs. Although no definitive data are available, there is the potential for slowing the use of additional technology, and the manpower needed to operate it. Decision making on technology usually remains in the institution, the institution being forced to make trade offs, unless the rate regulation mechanism allows increases to cover the costs of added technology. In some of the states with rate regulation, beds have been closed and limits placed on the quantity of certain technologies.

Medical necessity, as indicated earlier, is a concept that was part of private health insurance prior to Medicare and Medicaid. Until the creation of the NCHCT, decision making in both the public and private sector was random and ad hoc except for the routine exclusion of investigational drugs, devices, and procedures that were developing under biomedical research grants. The NCHCT was established in 1978, to coordinate technology assessment activities within the Department of Health and Human Services and to conduct assessments of the safety, effectiveness, cost effectiveness, social, economic and ethical issues related to technology. Its mandate was and is research and dissemination of information. Technology as defined in the law is:

> "....Any discrete and identifiable regimen or modality used to diagnose and treat illness, prevent disease, maintain patient well-being, or facili-

tate the provision of health care services."

The law and its interpretation clearly state that the Center cannot duplicate other activities and has no authority to regulate drugs, devices, treatment modalities nor does it have the authority to directly control the spread or phase out of technologies. The Center is also charged with stimulating the development and use of promising technologies.

The founders of the Center believed and still believe that there is a middle ground between a laissez faire attitude on technology and a rigid regulatory approach. The philosophy of the Center has been that the development of sound and systematic assessment and tools for assessment with broad public and private participation in the assessments and broad diffusion of the findings will lead to the voluntary use of the information by physicians, other health professionals, hospitals, third parties, and consumers, resulting in a more rational adoption and use of various technologies. In every activity undertaken by the Center, this philosophy was followed.

The NCHCT can and does have an indirect impact on Medicare decisions on reimbursement. The law requests the NCHCT make recommendations to the Secretary on laws administered by the Secretary. In conducting these assessments, the Center advertises the issue under consideration, widely solicits information from the public and the health professions, consults with other federal agencies like NIH or FDA which have particular expertise, and consults with private sector specialty societies. Public forums and conferences are also used to develop consensus in cooperation with NIH, FDA and the private sector. The conferences are planned by private sector interdisciplinary experts in the fields of medicine, economics, ethics, and consumers. The Center's activities are too new to evaluate in terms of the impact of its assessments and recent actions by the Reagan administration threaten the continuation of the Center's activities.

It is sometimes instructive to look at how other nations deal with similar problems, although their solutions are often not adaptable to our economic and social systems. In nations like Canada, Britain, Sweden and France, technology is controlled largely by limiting supply and through queueing mechanisms applied to elective procedures. Fixed budgets for hospitals and control of the number of special-

ists and consultants force allocation and technology decisions to be made explicitly by national and local communities and institutions. Yet these nations are also experiencing health care cost inflation in large part attributable
to advancing technology. While consumer expectations and
demand and physician demand for use of effective technology
clearly influence the introduction of new technology in
these nations, innovation often comes later and slower and
in planned, smaller quantities. A number of these nations
are discussing the establishment of programs like the NCHCT,
to assist in making rational decisions.

Our health care structure and the size and diversity of
our nation do not lend themselves to supply control and centralized budgeting. Competition may be an alternative, assuming that the theory behind competition will work. There
are several cautions, however. Competitive systems will
still need a mechanism to assess technology to be able to
make informed local and individual choices regarding technology and payment for technology by competing insurors or
delivery systems. Competition does have the potential for
controlling use rates, additive technologies and for selecting out ineffective technologies in health maintenance organization type operations. It also has the potential for
slowing the introduction of technology, but information on
technology is needed to make these decisions. However, consumer and physician pressures for the addition of technologies that _appear_ effective will continue and provider groups
may well compete on the basis of sophisticated technologies
resulting in ever escalating costs among all provider
groups. If the competition theories prove unsound, if tax
incentives and disincentives do not work as planned, or providers will not participate, and if we dismantle all planning and rate regulation, current cost escalation may look
modest in the future.

In my view, whether or not a competitive system devel-
ops, we cannot continue to approach the decision making process on technology mindlessly, by pure lottery, or what may
be worse, by not confronting choice at all. Too often in
the past serious social decisions have been made by indirectly avoiding the conflicts inherent in making choices.
Society has too often made these choices implicitly and by
happenstance. Who, for example, has gained and lost in the
decision to finance end stage renal disease through Medicare
at a cost exceeding $1 billion a year? What does the with-
holding of a technology or a slowing of the development of

a technology cost in lives, quality of life, productivity?

These are decisions that affect individuals, families, professionals, communities, and society as a whole. They affect scientific advances and allocation of resources for biomedical research; patterns of mortality, morbidity and disability; costs to individuals, employers, the government. The choices raise profound issues of social justice and the uses of public and private resources. In the future, as we continue to adjust our resource choices among different social and public goods, more and more, society will demand explicit consideration of the consequences of choices. If we do not want random, ill informed decisions on technology, some catalyst or convenor is needed to bring together all of the interests to regularly and systematically address the scientific, economic, social and ethical issues of medical technology. I believe the National Center for Health Care Technology could fill this function, whether we pursue the competition proposals or revert to regulatory approaches. In the absence of the Center and/or sufficient resources to fulfill its function, we will need to create some other mechanism in the private sector or we will continue to meet in conferences such as the Norfleet Forum to bemoan society's random, ill informed decisions, continued cost escalation, and the use or misuse of scarce resources.

The views presented in this paper are the views of the author and should not be construed as representing the views of the Association of Academic Health Centers.

REFERENCES

1.   U.S. Congress, House of Representatives, 95th Con-
     gress, 2nd Session, Report #95-1190 by the Committee
     on Interstate and Foreign Commerce: Health Services
     Research, Health Statistics and Health Care Technology
     Act, U.S.G.P.O. 1978, Washington, D.C.

REIMBURSEMENT FOR TECHNOLOGY: THE INSURER'S DILEMMA
H. Michael Schiffer

Introduction

Nostalgia is very fashionable right now--it always is in turbulent times. A lot of time and a lot of money are spent making new things look old and old things look better, and talking about the "good old days."

But when you get right down to taking a hard look at the good old days, sometimes you find that they were not all that good. Certainly this is true in health care. We all recognize that there are still many areas in which chicken soup and a pat on the back do as much or more good as the best that medical science and technology have to offer. But let's face it--the good old days in medicine when the family general practitioner was the family friend, were also the days when kids died of polio and women died in childbirth. The good old days were also the days of the dual standard of care--which all too often meant no care for some people.

But progress has its price. And if progress in medicine is technology and increased access, its price has been increased costs and a certain amount of commercializing and depersonalizing of the health care transaction. It seems to me that as a society we have elected to pay that price. But I believe that there is a limit to what we will pay and that we are approaching that limit.

The technology issue is of great interest to me in itself. As an illustration of some fundamental problems in the health care system and of the constraints group health insurers face in operating within the system, I think it is even more important.

Technology and Health Care Costs

I would like to make the point--almost trite by now--that medical technology is more than medical hardware. In the broadest sense, technology is applied knowledge. The Office of Technology Assessment has defined medical technology as "procedures, drugs, equipment and services combining these elements used in the practice of medicine." So technology is nuclear magnetic resonance and cardiac imaging, but it is also coronary artery bypass surgery and drugs used to treat heart problems without surgery. It is medical practice itself.

Although our health care system has a number of limitations, I would hope that everyone could agree on two premises. First, that the U.S. health care system--whatever its problems--is far preferable to what anyone else has, at least partly because of its level of technology. Second, the most pressing problem now facing that system is health care cost inflation which if left unchecked stands a chance of bringing the system down around us.

Until recently, technology has been the whipping boy of the health care cost debate. Enormous resources have been poured into what have turned out to be snipe hunts--quests for "the culprit" behind rising health care costs--be it CT scanners, profit-making delivery organizations, overinsurance, lack of competition or something else. Now we are moving into the second and third generation of fabulously sophisticated and expensive technological equipment. The question is "will we persist in this futile strategy?" Will we continue our search for a scapegoat for the cost inflation problem that may make us feel better, but in the final analysis does nothing about the problem itself? I hope not. And, I think, based upon what I have heard so far at this conference, that we are more forward thinking. We are less likely to be led astray by red herrings--whether they are called nuclear magnetic resonance, cardiac imaging or something else.

The basic question seems to be how do we control what we pay given the level of technological quality we have come to expect. Now I am all too familiar with the role insurance has played in contributing to cost increases. The theory is that "rich" insurance plans negate consumer and provider interest in costs. And it is true that plans with low deductibles, low coinsurance and high first dollar coverage have been a problem. I think we have to keep in mind though that the push for greater first dollar coverage is at this point coming from the consumer. We are working to increase buyer awareness about what plan features are in their best interest from a cost standpoint and hope that demand for this type of coverage will increase. Talk about the elimination of the insurance function, however, begs the question. I think few of us would be willing to live with the social dislocations that would result from the elimination of the health insurance function. The problem is not insurance per se, any more than it is technology per se. The problem is the incentive structure that is part and parcel of today's retrospective, cost-based reimbursement system.

Whether retrospective cost-based reimbursement originated with a private third party payer--in this case Blue Cross--or with the provider community is irrelevant. The point is it has become a determining factor in all major cost-generating decisions in health care--including the adoption and use of health care technology. It has allowed the decision makers to avoid uncomfortable "trade-offs." After all, why should we make trade-offs if we can have everything? But can we continue to have everything indefinitely? I think we cannot. And I think the signs that we are approaching the limits of what we can do are right in front of us.

Evidence is mounting that the health care industry is in for some lean years. The era of health care expansion ushered in by Medicare and Medicaid in 1965 is drawing to a close. About 40 percent of health care expenditures are financed by Medicare and Medicaid, but the federal government is searching for ways to limit its share of health expenditures--or at least to constrain further growth.

For several years now they have sought to control Medicare expenditures through increasingly strict regulations promulgated under Section 223 of the Medicare and Medicaid Amendments. We have moved from a time when Section 223 covered routine costs of about 300 hospitals to where they sweep in close to 20 percent. In the words of one observer of government health financing, the federal establishment is approaching the point where they will pay up to but not over the average cost of caring for a Medicare beneficiary. Current administration proposals include expanding Section 223 to cover ancillary as well as routine costs, publication of

a list of reasonable physician fees, and restricting reimbursement for radiologists and pathologists.

It is clear that there will be further restrictions in
government reimbursement although perhaps not those currently proposed. The question for the health care industry
then is even more basic than "what will be the source of
funding for new technology?" The question is where will we
get the funds to sustain even the present generation of
technology?

The Cost Shift Phenomenon

There is an easy answer to this question and that is that we
will get the funds from the private sector. Let me suggest
why this is a dangerous route. In hospital care alone the
private sector is subsidizing public patients to the tune of
almost $5 billion a year and that number is going steadily
upward. Since 1972 the federal government has systematically controlled its expenditures by shifting costs to private
patients. The cost shift phenomenon has become a hidden
tax of major proportions. Among the hospital costs not
recognized by the Medicare program are bad debt and chari-
ty care, certain equity capital requirements for replacement
of assets, and some education and research costs. Between
1975 and 1979 the "differential" or shortfall between hospital
costs and government reimbursement rose from $12 to $41
per adjusted patient day as depicted in Figure 1. If this
rate of growth is sustained, the differential will reach $99
per adjusted patient day in 1983. Although the private
sector may be the "deep pocket" in this case, we are not
bottomless. The ability of insurers to pass through cost
increases to our corporate clients is not, as some think,
limitless. We are witnessing a new corporate militancy about
hospital costs.

The Private Health Insurance Market

The question is "what can private health insurers do about
health care costs?" A few words about the private health
insurance market are probably in order at this point. I
would like to clear up two popular misconceptions. First
is that health insurance is a "loss leader." Major insurers
for whom health insurance is a billion dollar line of business cannot afford to operate it as a loss. Second is that
private health insurers possess and exercise vast market
power. The private health insurance industry is usually

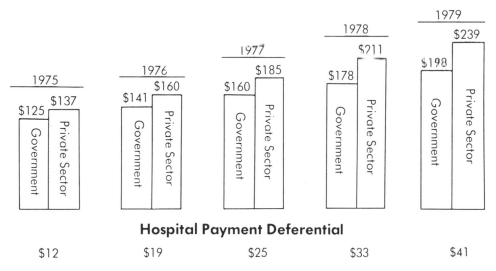

Hospital Payment Deferential

Figure 1. 1975 to 1979, Short term hospital average payments per adjusted patient day by government and by private sector patients divided into two segments--the commercial carriers and Blue Cross/Blue Shield. There are over 700 commercial insurance carriers, no one of which controls more than five percent of a given health care market. The 112 Blue Cross/Blue Shield plans, on the other hand, collectively control about 50 percent of the market. So the commercial insurers are in no position--the antitrust laws being what they are--to control costs directly through negotiations with providers.

The Insurer's Role Vis-a-Vis Technology

As to the relation of the technology issue to private health insurers, two questions need to be raised. First, what can or should insurers do about health care technology? Second, what can insurers do about the reimbursement system that fosters the uncritical adoption and utilization of health care technology?

Protection against the large, infrequently occurring loss is what insurance is all about. So from this standpoint, CT scans, bypass surgery and other "big ticket" technologies are ideal candidates for insurance reimbursement. But technology presents a special dilemma for group health insurers. On the one hand, cost containment argues against the coverage of expensive possibly unproven procedures which are not completely substitutable for their predecessors. On the other hand, pressures from employees are likely to be reflected by employer demands for coverage of new procedures. The last point is key. Sometimes it is forgotten that health insurance is an "employee benefit" designed to supplement wages and relieve the employer of financial worries about cost of health care for workers and their families. Over 80 percent of health insurance is written on a group basis. And employers like to be on the leading edge of doing good things for their people.

This brings me to a paradox that is a fact of life for those in the group health insurance business. Employers as a group are increasingly concerned and vocal about health care costs. Witness the strength of the Washington Business Group on Health. Individually they are concerned about the cost of health insurance. Witness the trend toward self-insured or partially self-insured plans. But try to sell a plan change that has even the appearance of reducing coverage, and you run into a brick wall.

Some have challenged insurers to resist "traveling with

the herd." They have argued, for example, for abolition of usual, customary and reasonable (UCR) reimbursement for surgeons. In the days before high inflation, UCR was a valid concept. It kept the benefit plan up-to-date with a minimum of administrative expense. It is a concept that is deeply ingrained and I would like to suggest why it will not easily be abandoned despite its flaws. The market for group health insurance is a very competitive one in which the large employer calls the tune. Benefit structures are not determined unilaterally by the insurer. Far from it. An insurer who refused a client's demands for coverage of a new technology or who decided to switch to a more restrictive reimbursement methodology would find his place taken rather quickly by a competitor. And antitrust laws prohibit joint insurer decision making regarding products and rates. We cannot decide together not to cover a new piece of medical technology or change our method of reimbursement, and we are unlikely to stick our necks out and make that decision alone.

Is this wrong? With respect to technology I am not at all sure that it is. For one thing, individual carriers have no expertise on which to assess health care technology. And I am unaware of the existence of any independent agency capable of making assessments within a time frame that would help us. Once the decisions come out, we have already been operating on our own policy for months, sometimes years. So any insurer decision would be made on a strictly "best guess" basis. For the most part, group insurers are swept along on the tide of prevailing medical opinion. I am not sure that private health insurance should call the shots on what kind of treatment people do or do not get. Certainly no one has given us the authority to do this and our customers have not asked us to do it. There is a fundamental philosophical question about whether it is in the public interest to put a private industry in what amounts to a regulatory posture. If public safety and welfare is truly at stake, then it seems to me government must control the associated problems and do so in a timely fashion. If quality of care and comfort of the patients are at stake, then the medical profession should participate.

So this is the bad news. The good news is that I believe private health insurers, not acting alone or as an industry, but acting in conjunction with all of the concerned parties, can do a great deal about the reimbursement system. Retrospective cost-based reimbursement need not take us into the 21st century. In fact, if it lasts that long the health care system may not make it to the 21st century. The Omnibus Budget Reconciliation Act calls for the development of a prospective payment system for Medicare.

The Diagnostic Related Group (DRG) experiment in New Jersey is a sign of things to come. Although it is not perfect, the DRG approach offers several advantages over the current system. For one thing, it forces providers to consider the costs of decisions to order ancillary services, adopt new technologies or prolong hospital stays. Another advantage is that it brings about greater equity among classes of payors. The federal government is now developing a DRG based system for Medicare reimbursement and hopes to have it operating in three years. I am also in favor of prospective hospital reimbursement as it has been employed by a few hospital cost commissions and would be interested in private sector initiatives in reimbursement reforms as well. What I do <u>not</u> regard as useful, at least at this point, are proposals to control costs solely by controlling the adoption of technology through state and federal regulatory agencies or through private sector voluntary efforts at self-regulation, without addressing reimbursement incentives. This amounts to what Lewis Thomas might call "halfway" technology to deal with "half-way" technology.

Those of us who have a stake in our health care system--providers, payers, consumers and regulators--have an obligation not to stand by and watch the system fall of its own weight while we take profits, or consolidate power, or maximize utility, or whatever the appropriate jargon is. Parochial interests have to be pushed far enough into the background to enable us to join together in a ground-up restructuring of reimbursement. It is my hope that we can build something that, in the process of making each of the players a little less comfortable, will increase the long run stability of the system as a whole. This is the fundamental challenge that faces us in an era of contracting government responsibility. If we decline to meet it, we cannot complain about what is imposed on us as a result.

ALLOCATING RESOURCES
FOR HEALTH
J. Michael McGinnis, M.D.

This paper begins by providing a little perspective, through a few cases, which are short but contain important lessons.

1. John Clark was a 52 year old white male salesman who presented to the hospital for examination because of weight loss and shortness of breath. He had a history of smoking two packs of cigarettes per day for 33 years. A chest x-ray revealed a large mass in the upper lobe of the left lung. Bronchoscopy and biopsy indicated bronchogenic carcinoma--lung cancer. Mr. Clark died six months later, leaving a wife and three teenage children.

2. Sarah Fargo was a 29 year old black female who came to the hospital because of a nosebleed that would not stop. Mrs. Fargo had been having nosebleeds and headaches intermittently over the previous several months, and had also noticed a sudden deterioration in the vision in her right eye. On admission, her blood pressure was 230/180. Admission blood tests revealed severe kidney impairment, and she ultimately went on to total renal shutdown, requiring dialysis, bilateral nephroctomy and cadaver transplant.

3. Emery Phillips was a jovial 63 year old white male construction worker who had brought his ailing sister to the emergency room for treatment of a long-standing heart condition.

143

While awaiting her disposition, Mr. Phillips was approached by a hospital attendant who remarked about his labored breathing and suggested he consider a chest x-ray. Thirty minutes later a large mass was detected at the lower lobe of his right lung. Mr. Phillips was admitted to the hospital for an extensive diagnostic workup, ultimately including thoracotomy and biopsy of the mass. Diagnosis: mesothelioma--a highly malignant tumor associated with exposure to asbestos. Mr. Phillips' only known exposure to asbestos had been 27 years earlier when he had helped install asbestos-containing insulation on a job. The tumor rapidly spread, and four months later Emery Phillips died.

4.   George Edwards was a 47 year old white male high school teacher who presented to the emergency room with acute onset of chest pain radiating down his left arm. An EKG suggested a subendocardial infarct. Mr. Edwards had a two year history of mild hypertension, about 140/95, one pack per day smoking for 20 years, and a blood cholesterol level between 260 and 280. Twenty-four hours after admission, Mr. Edwards suffered a cardiac arrest, was resuscitated, stabilized with a cardiac pacemaker, regained consciousness after 15 hours, and left the hospital 22 days later for a home rehabilitation program.

5.   Rana Mishra was a three month old girl from a tiny Indian village of 200 people about 150 miles east of New Delhi on the Ganges Plain. On first observation by the World Health Organization team, she had a high fever, was breathing with difficulty, and was covered on the hands, feet and face with large fluid-filled pustules. She died of smallpox 24 hours later.

These people were real people with real problems. Under different names, they were all patients of mine, just a decade ago--even less for the Indian baby--and all had courses of illness typical for the disease and the location.

The important thing is <u>not</u> that these were great human tragedies, which they obviously were, but that medical progress in just one short decade has been dramatic.

o   John Clark died of lung cancer because he had smoked two packs of cigarettes a day for over 30 years. But from 1964 to 1979 the share of white males who smoke dropped from 54 percent to about 36 percent.

o   Sarah Fargo lost her kidneys, and most of the vision in one eye, because she suffered from long-standing and undiagnosed high blood pressure. Today, though the data are still being collected, it seems likely that the share of people whose blood pressure is under control has substantially more than doubled in the last decade. And, most importantly, stroke deaths declined by 40 percent in the decade from 1970 to 1980.

o   Emery Phillips died of a mesothelioma because he had been exposed to asbestos nearly 30 years earlier. Reports of the health threats of asbestos have appeared in scientific literature since the turn of the century, but until recently very little has been done.

     Today, however, vigilance with respect to asbestos containing products is much more prevalent, and the general public is much more aware of the dangers. A momentum is developing.

o   George Edwards very nearly died of atherosclerotic heart disease. He was the classic heart patient identified for us by a 15 year study in Framingham Union High School District. Today people are smoking less, their blood pressure is better controlled, and they are exercising more and eating less saturated fat and cholesterol. And heart disease deaths dropped by 25 percent in the decade from 1970 to 1980.

o   Rana Mishra died of smallpox, a disease which has probably taken more human lives throughout history than any other disease known to man. Yet, as of 1977, smallpox has been eradicated from the face of the earth, the first disease which man has ever deliberately eliminated as a threat.

The trends I have described for you ought to be encouraging, especially for Americans.

We are emerging from a remarkable generation--indeed a remarkable decade--for health in this country.

Biomedical research has been unfolding the mysteries of the gene, and putting the lessons into motion for use in clinical care. New diagnostic technology allows us to peer into the cellular nooks and crannies of the human organism.

But has something else been noticed?

It was prevention--and not the application of expensive technology to diagnosis and treatment of disease--that has yielded the lion's share of these gains.

Technology has yielded virtually no gains in the prospects for lung cancer patients. Yet, due to the dramatic shift in the attitudes and behavior towards smoking, a downturn is expected to begin in lung cancer deaths over the next 10 to 15 years.

Considerable resources have been devoted to sophisticated technology for diagnosing and monitoring heart disease. Mr. Edwards is alive today as a result of some of that technology. Yet much--indeed the consensus would argue, most--of the gains against heart disease in the last decade have occurred as a result of simple shifts in behavior: reduced consumption of fatty foods; reduced smoking; more exercise; better adherence to antihypertensive regimens.

Likewise, in high blood pressure control there have been no quantum technologic leaps in the last decade. The sphygmomanometer is the same as its been for years. For the most part, the medications are variations on the same theme. But physicians and patients alike have been made more aware of the problem--and stroke deaths are down 40 percent.

With smallpox eradication, clearly technology played a role in the production and refinement of vaccine. A reasonably good vaccination procedure has been available since Edward Jenner observed the protective nature of cowpox infection in 1798. But, the two dominant features of the successful final years of the eradication program were the use of the tiny bifurcated vaccination needle, which cost a fraction of a cent and could greatly facilitate the vaccination process, and the emphasis on the strategy of surveillance and localized containment.

In fact the gains in prevention over the last decade have been so substantial that several powerful myths have been laid to rest, myths that have persisted in some respects for centuries, about our control (or lack of control) over disease:

1.   The myth that no disease can be entirely eliminated.

--Yet, the smallpox virus now exists only in four laboratories around the world.

2.   The myth that all chronic diseases are inevitable consequences of the aging process.

--Yet, heart disease and stroke, the leading killers of Americans, have had an unprecedented decline in the last 10 years.

3.   The myth that your physician is the person most important to your health.

--When we are ill, our physicians are very important indeed.

--But if we are well, as most of us are, each of us has the greatest opportunity to determine our own health destiny.

The latter point is borne out by an analysis of the Center for Disease Control estimating the relative contributions of the factors involved in reducing premature mortality for the 10 leading causes of death. If you divide those factors into four groups (environmental, hereditary, lifestyle, and medical services), the relative contributions of each are estimated to look something like the following:

o   Environmental factors account for about 20 percent of the capability to reduce premature death.

o   Hereditary factors account for another 20 percent.

o   Lifestyle factors--those over which each person has direct control--account for about 50 percent.

o   And medical services account for only about 10 percent.

At this point, technology effectively contributes to interventions only in the latter category.

It can be viewed in another way. About 9.4 percent of the Gross National Product (GNP) of the United States is spent for health care. If all of the GNP were spent for medical services to treat disease, only about 10 percent of the premature deaths would be affected. The implication is not that most technologies are of essentially no use in affecting health status. Many, of course, have applications at which one can only marvel in certain clinical situations. One need only look at the gains with respect to neonatal intensive care to recognize this.

But a sense of balance is required. Particularly in times of shrinking resouces, as we set about the allocation of those resources, two prominent issues must be considered:

o   First, Americans must be aware of the limitations of technology--especially diagnostic technology-- in affecting the national health profile;

o   Second, Americans must acknowledge the relative prospects for prevention as a contributor to health gains.

With regards to the limitations of technology, it should be recalled that for the most part, medical technologies are devoted to detection of illness or physiologic aberrations--not to interventions.

The vast majority of new technologies which drive up the costs of hospitalizations are devoted to making measurements of bodily conditions or processes, rather than changing those processes. As such, they really operate at the margins of genuine clinical progress. But, because of the complexity and mystique of many of these instruments, it is tempting to conclude that they must surely be doing wonderful things to improve the clinical course of events.

Herein lies an important flaw in our view: too frequently science is confused with technology. In effect, technology becomes science and inherits an extraordinary degree of tolerance. In fact, many technologies represent, not extensions of the search for new understanding through careful implementation of the scientific method; rather, they represent the premature application to clinical problems of selected scientific insights without adequate prior understanding of the consequences.

The philosophy seems to be that if a technologic innovation can enhance the predictive value of a positive test even a few percentage points, then that innovation must surely be adopted and apparently at any price. As a result, society is burdened with incremental expenses, incurred with each new iteration of an apparatus, which can far outstrip the incremental utility in terms of health outcome.

The condition is one of illusory benefits and real costs. And the condition seems to be intractable. As long as current methods are operative for introduction and diffusion of new technologies in clinical medicine, there is no indication that greater efficiencies in terms of improved health status per unit cost are soon to be forthcoming.

A direct consequence of the tremendous drain on our resources from the inefficient diffusion of both diagnostic, and to some extent, interventive technologies, is a squeezing of our ability to support preventive interventions. This is so in spite of the fact that the vast share of the capability to alter premature death lies outside the realm of clinical medicine.

Part of the reason for the constraint on preventive activities relates to the paucity of residual resources. But part also is attributable to the strict criteria applied to preventive measures, before their introduction. It is ironic that the health impact assessments which are virtually non-existent as a precondition for deployment of most clinical technologies related to disease management, are imposed so strictly on questions of paying for measures of disease prevention.

I happen to be one who favors rigorous accountability criteria, but I am struck by the contrast in the way in which society parcels out its resources.

Nonetheless, with respect to prevention, the prospects for large gains from small investments seem quite good. For adults, there is every reason to believe that heart disease and stroke death rates will continue to decline, as people continue to pay closer attention to healthy behavior.

For children, there is every reason to believe that sustained vigilance will cause the incidence of the vaccine-preventable diseases of childhood to continue to fall. We may in fact be within months of eliminating measles as an indigenous problem in this country. And we ought also to anticipate that fluoridation of local water supplies will continue to reduce the most common and one of the most expensive health problems: dental caries.

For infants, through improved prenatal care and habits and enhanced access to regional perinatal care, we ought to anticipate attaining a 35 percent reduction in infant mortality, to below a level of nine deaths per 1000 live births by 1990. And we ought not to forget that there are a number of technologies on the horizon whose potential applications to prevention make the next decade or two particularly tantalizing.

For example, with the advent of recombinant DNA technology, there is the prospect of antenatal repair of genetic defects. Many inherited errors of metabolism are the result of simple problems with complex effects. That is, a solitary change in a nucleotide base of a DNA molecule, may result in a defect in the production of a single enzyme which may control very important metabolic processes.

It is possible that through recombinant DNA technology we will eventually have the skill to repair that defect, and plug a physiologic hole in the process of an individual's developmental capabilities.

Another emerging technology of potential import to the national health lies in the production of hybridomas and monoclonal antibodies. While the terminology sounds like something out of Jules Verne, the concept is really very simple.

We are, in effect, on the verge of being able to use physiologic processes to produce, in mass quantities, agents--antibodies--which have the ability to fix very precisely and selectively to targeted chemical structures. The potential applications of this process are vast: ranging from improved diagnostics, to bolstered immune systems, cancer control, and even cleaning up oil spills.

Finally, possibly the most exciting prospective scientific development lies with the set of advances that can be expected with respect to the neurosciences. This field, with all its implications for health and behavior, is quite simply booming.

Historically the scientific pursuit of knowledge in the fields of biology and behavior have gone down separate paths.   With new discoveries in the last decade about the brain's circuits and the brain's chemistry, this distinction between behavior and biology is beginning to break down.

Perhaps the most striking discoveries have been those related to the role of peptides as neurotransmitters. Neurotransmitters are those substances found in the nervous system which are released on depolarization of a nerve cell and provide chemical links between nerve cells in the transmission of electrical impulses from one cell to the next. They are, therefore, the links through which all behavior is mediated or, at least, modulated.

A generation ago very little was known about any neurotransmitters and then, through the 1960s, a few amines were the only well-recognized transmitters--norepinephrine, acetylcholine, and serotonin. The last decade though, has seen an explosion in the number of identifiable neurotransmitters--now about two dozen, but possibly more than 200.

To date the most publicized of the neuropeptide transmitters are the endorphins--targeted to opiate receptors-- found concentrated in circuits controlling brain centers for cardiovascular, endocrine and autonomic activity. These neurochemicals are linked to various facets of a wide range of physiologic and psychological functions, including emotional responses, motivation, sexual behavior, sleep, apetite, alertness, pain relief, sense of well-being, and learning and memory.

An important feature of neuropeptides is their sustained action over time. Unlike our conventional understanding of the instantaneous release and retrieval of neurotransmitters, the neuropeptides may persist at the brain receptor site for minutes or hours. Their presence then modulates the flow of information within the brain, and between the brain and the endocrine system, the central nervous system's link to the other systems of the human organism.

Specifically, it has been found that certain of these peptides are released in the brain, then travel to the anterior pituitary, and out to the rest of the body.

Through our studies, in addition to beginning to gain a better understanding of the biochemical nature of mood, attitude and behavior, some clues about factors involved in controlling the release of these transmitters are being gleaned. As these clues take better shape the potential for their regulation may be gained not only through exogenous means, but possibly endogenously as well through alteration of behavioral patterns involved in the physiologic feedback loop.

We can only speculate at this point about the ultimate outcomes of these forays into the molecular structure of a man's motives, but the implications for health promotion-- and for enhanced sense of well-being--are staggering.

Each of these prospective developments indicates that history is unfolding as a set of great compounding experiences. That is to say, it is progressing not in an orderly linear fashion--one event spaced neatly after another--but exponentially: a series of reinforcing developments whose rate of occurrence constantly confounds human anticipation.

As a result, predicting the future, with respect to technology or anything else, is something to be approached only with great caution.

One thing is very clear. This is, that very potent forces are at work to create new demands on our capability to improve health.

First, demography is beginning to make itself known very prominently on the health agenda. Americans are an aging population. And while all chronic diseases need not be inevitable consequences of the aging process, a greater share of those conditions will occur. This implies a shift in the types of demands for medical care, more attention to long-term care and rehabilitation--and more costs.

Second, there is a certain uneasiness toward the other end of the life spectrum--with adolescents and young adults. Our young people seem to bear a disproportionate share of our contemporary social ills. They are, for example, the only age group for which the death rate has actually increased in the last 20 years. And the problems of violence--suicide, homicide and motor vehicle accidents--which afflict young people are problems for which there are no easy answers. Yet they are problems which demand more attention and more resources.

Third, for progress in health to continue, behavior change becomes a larger and larger factor--and it is clearly the most difficult of measures to assure. Though there has been a 20 percent drop in smoking, a 10 to 15 percent reduction in the consumption of fatty foods, and a boom in exercise over the last 15 years, the profiles of drug and alcohol abuse have worsened. And there is no guarantee that the gains seen have not occurred among those most easily recruited to change rather than among the most vulnerable. A sustained effort is needed to capture the gains possible.

Finally, to echo a theme raised earlier by Dr. Joseph, our world is becoming ever smaller and ever more interdependent. As a result, there is no choice but to be cognizant of the global factors which shape the attitudes, capabilities and conditions of our neighbors. The health and nutritional needs in many parts of the world are awesome and growing. It is necessary--and it is inevitable--that Americans will become fuller participants in the struggle against these problems.

Each of the trends mentioned holds the prospect of requiring substantial resources. And each underscores the need to ensure that investments yield worthy and reasonable returns. Unproductive--and even frivolous--costs which drain precious resources at a time when the case for alternative uses of those resources is becoming so compelling cannot be tolerated.

We have an important obligation to ensure that our substantial resources are not used to build a technologic monument to inefficiency.

I would like to close with a quote from Henry George of more than 100 years ago. It was intended to apply to more purely political processes, but I think is relevant for the theme of this forum. It reads as follows:

> "So long as all the increased wealth which modern progress brings, goes but to build up inequities and inefficiencies, to increase luxury and make sharper the contrast between the House of Have and the House of Want, progress is not real and cannot be permanent."

We still have the opportunity to alter the course of events. We must be sure we have the will.

APPENDIX A:
Forum Trustees and University President

For The University of Tennessee
Center for the Health Sciences:

James R. Gay, M.D., Norfleet Forum Director and
Director of Special Programs

James C. Hunt, M.D.
Vice President for Health Affairs and Chancellor

Bland W. Cannon, M.D.
Special Advisor for Professional Affairs

Stephen T. Miller, M.D.
Associate Professor of Community Medicine

For the Memphis-Plough Community Foundation:

George M. Houston
Chairman of the Board
Mid-South Title Insurance Company
Memphis, Tennessee

Edward W. Reed, M.D.
General Surgery
Memphis, Tennessee

University President:

Edward J. Boling, Ph.D.
President
The University of Tennessee
Knoxville, Tennessee

155